KETO DIET

THE COMPLETE KETO DIET COOKBOOK FOR MEN AND WOMEN OVER 50. LEARN HOW TO LOSE WEIGHT AND BURN FAT EASILY WITH A 30-DAY MEAL PLAN. QUICK RECIPES FOR YOUR PREPARATIONS

ROSE CHILD

Table of Contents

INTRODUCTION 6

THE KETOGENIC DIET BASICS 9

- What is the Ketogenic Diet 9
- Getting into Ketosis 10
- When I am in Ketosis 11
- Benefits of Ketogenic Diet 12
- Keto Diet FAQs 14
- Keto Grocery List 17

KETOGENIC DIET FOR MEN AND WOMEN OVER 50 18

- The relationship between Aging and Nutritional Need 18
- How Proper Nutrition Helps Slow Down Aging 22
- Tips and Tricks to be Learnt about Keto Diet For Seniors 24
- Tips on Maintaining Ketosis For Senior Over 50 27
- Food to Avoid 27

30-DAY MEAL PLAN FOR PEOPLE OVER 50 29

- 30-Day Meal Plan Sample 29

KETO BREAKFAST RECIPES 32

1. Almond Coconut Egg Wraps 32
2. Bacon & Avocado Omelet 32
3. Bacon & Cheese Frittata . 33
4. Bacon & Egg Breakfast Muffins 34
5. Bacon Hash 34
6. Bagels With Cheese 35
7. Baked Apples 36
8. Baked Eggs In The Avocado 36
9. Banana Pancakes 37
10. Breakfast Skillet 37
11. Brunch BLT Wrap 38
12. Cheesy Bacon & Egg Cups 38
13. Coconut Keto Porridge ... 39
14. Cream Cheese Eggs 40
15. Creamy Basil Baked Sausage 40

KETO BREAD RECIPES 42

16. Holiday Morning Bread .. 42
17. Masterpiece Bread 43
18. Dense Morning Bread 44
19. Multi Seeds Bread 45
20. Sandwich Bread 46
21. Magic Cheese Bread......... 47
22. 10-Minutes Bread 48
23. Subtle Rosemary Bread ... 49
24. Brunch Time Bread.......... 50
25. Amazing Cheddar Bread .. 51

KETO VEGETABLES RECIPES 53

26. Grain-Free Creamy Noodles 53
27. Meat-Free Zoodles Stroganoff................................ 54
28. Eye-Catching Veggies....... 55
29. Favorite Punjabi Curry.... 56
30. Traditional Indian Curry . 57
31. Vinegar Braised Cabbage . 58
32. Green Veggies Curry......... 58
33. Fuss-Free Veggies Bake 59
34. 4 Veggies Combo 60
35. Midweek Veggie Supper ... 61
36. Buttery Veggies............... 62
37. Best Tasting Kabobs 63

KETO SOUP & STEW RECIPES 65

38. Winter Comfort stew 65
39. Ideal Cold Weather Stew 66
40. Weekend Dinner Stew....... 67
41. Mexican Pork Stew 68
42. Hungarian Pork Stew...... 69
43. Yellow Chicken Soup 70

44. Curry Soup 72
45. Delicious Tomato Basil Soup 73
46. Chicken Enchilada Soup ... 74
47. Buffalo Chicken Soup 75
48. Slow Cooker Taco Soup ... 76
49. Wedding Soup 77
50. Slow Cooker Taco Soup ... 78

KETO SNACK RECIPES 80

51. Keto Fat Bombs 80
52. Asparagus Fries with Dipping Sauce 81
53. Bacon-Wrapped Jalapeño Poppers 82
54. Pumpkin Roll Fat Bombs .. 82
55. Smoked Salmon Dip 84
56. Chewy Granola Bars 84
57. Almond Butter Fudge Bars 85
58. Creamed Spinach Pockets with Apple Slaw 87
59. No-Churn Ice Cream 88
60. Cheesecake Cupcakes 89
61. Brownies 90
62. Chocolate Peanut Butter Cups 91
63. Peanut Butter Cookies 91
64. Low-Carb Almond Coconut Sandies 92
65. Creme Brulee 93

KETO SALAD RECIPES 95

66. Chicken avocado salad 95
67. Low carb Caesar salad 96
68. Keto broccoli salad 97
69. Keto chicken-cheese salad 98
70. Keto hamburger salad 98
71. Keto tomato and avocado salad 99
72. Calamari mayo with cauliflower broccoli salad 100
73. Chicken Spinach salad 101

KETO RED MEAT RECIPES 102

74. Classic Pork Tenderloin 102
75. Signature Italian Pork Dish 103
76. Flavor Packed Pork Loin 104
77. Spiced Pork Tenderloin . 105
78. Sticky Pork Ribs 106
79. Valentine's Day Dinner . 107
80. South East Asian Steak Platter 108
81. Pesto Flavored Steak 109
82. Flawless Grilled Steak .. 110
83. Mongolian Beef 111
84. Sicilian Steak Pinwheel.. 112
85. American Beef Wellington 113
86. Pastry-Free Beef Wellington 114

KETO FISH & SEAFOOD RECIPES 116

87. Super Salmon Parcel 116
88. New England Salmon Pie 117
89. Juicy Garlic Butter Shrimp 118
90. Simple Lemon Garlic Shrimp 119
91. Flavorful Shrimp Creole 119
92. Creamy Scallops 120
93. Perfect Pan-Seared Scallops 121
94. Easy Baked Shrimp Scampi 121
95. Delicious Blackened Shrimp 122
96. Creamy Parmesan Shrimp 122
97. Pan Fry Shrimp & Zucchini 123

KETO SAUCES & DRESSINGS RECIPES 125

98. AMERICAN JACK DANIEL'S SAUCE (KETO VERSION) 125
99. FRESH MUSHROOM SAUCE 126
100. SPICY CITRUS BBQ SAUCE 126
101. ITALIAN PESTO DIP WITH GROUND ALMONDS 127
102. KETO "CHIMICHURRI" SAUCE 128

KETO SMOOTHIES RECIPES 129

103. PEANUT BUTTER CUP SMOOTHIE 129
104. BERRY GREEN SMOOTHIE 129
105. LEMON-CASHEW SMOOTHIE 130
106. SPINACH-BLUEBERRY SMOOTHIE 131
107. CREAMY CINNAMON SMOOTHIE 131

KETO VEGAN RECIPES 132

108. CHOCOLATE SEA SALT SMOOTHIE 132
109. EGGPLANT LASAGNA 132
110. KETO VEGAN CAULIFLOWER AND TOFU STIR FRY 133
111. KETO VEGAN CURRY 134
112. SHIRATAKI NOODLES WITH VEGAN ALFREDO SAUCE 135

KETO CHAFFLE RECIPES 137

113. PEANUT CHAFFLES 137
114. GRILLED CHEESE CHAFFLE 137
115. BAKED POTATO CHAFFLE USING JICAMA 138
116. BREAKFAST CHAFFLE SANDWICH 139
117. PEANUT BUTTER AND JELLY CHAFFLES 140
118. HALLOUMI CHEESE CHAFFLES 141
119. CHAFFLES BENEDICT 141
120. EGGNOG CHAFFLES 142
121. BLUE CHEESE CHAFFLE BITES 143
122. CHAFFLE FRUIT SNACKS . 144
123. KETO BELGIAN SUGAR CHAFFLES 145

KETO DESSERT RECIPES 146

124. NO-BAKE CHOCOLATE "OATMEAL" BARS 146
125. NO-BAKE PEANUT BUTTER CARAMEL COOKIES 147
126. SUGAR COOKIE BARS 148
127. DAIRY-FREE PEANUT BUTTER BARS 149
128. VANILLA BEAN SEMIFREDDO 150

CONCLUSION 152

Introduction

The ketogenic diet, which is more popularly known as the keto diet, is a type of eating plan which includes fat-rich and low-carbohydrate foods. For centuries, this diet has been used in the treatment of a number of medical conditions. For instance, back in the nineteenth century, the keto diet was commonly recommended to those suffering from diabetes to help manage their condition. In the year 1920, experts had introduced this diet as an effective treatment for children who have epilepsy, especially for those who didn't respond well to medications. Because of the potential health benefits of the diet, it has been used and studied in closely monitored environments for the treatment of other conditions, such as brain-related diseases, heart disease, polycystic ovary syndrome, inflammation, and cancer.

Apart from these health benefits, the keto diet is also getting a lot of positive attention as an effective strategy for weight loss. This is because of the low-carb diet trend, which began back in the 1970s with the Atkins diet. The Atkins diet is a high-protein, low-carb diet. Back then, this diet became a huge commercial success. It also brought low-carb dieting to a whole new level. Now, it seems like the keto diet is taking center stage and for a good reason.

How Does It Work?

Basically, the principle behind the keto diet is that when you follow it, you're depriving your body of glucose, which just happens to be the main energy source of all the body's cells. Normally, glucose comes from foods that contain carbohydrates. While on the diet, your body will produce an alternative type of fuel source known as ketones, which come from your body's stored fats.

Out of all the parts in our body, the brain demands the most and the steadiest supply of glucose because it's unable to store glucose. But when you eat minimal amounts of carbohydrates, your body will acquire your glucose stores from your liver. Then it will temporarily break down muscles to release that glucose. If you keep on following the same diet for about three to four days and your body uses up the stored glucose, then your insulin blood levels will start to decrease.

When this happens, your body will start using fat as its primary fuel source. The liver will start producing ketones from the fat stores, which your body then uses when there is no glucose. As ketone bodies build up in your blood, you enter a metabolic state known as ketosis. Unlike when you fast for long periods, following the keto diet carefully ensures that your ketone blood levels won't reach harmful levels, which, in turn, might result in ketoacidosis.

Diabetic ketoacidosis, or simply ketoacidosis, is a serious medical condition that occurs as one of the complications of diabetes. This condition causes high levels of blood sugar as well as the accumulation of ketones in the body, raising the acidity of the blood. This condition may also develop when your body doesn't have adequate levels of insulin, so it begins to burn fat for fuel. Ketoacidosis is a life-threatening condition. It's important to follow the keto diet properly so you can achieve ketosis but won't go so far that you develop ketoacidosis. How soon your body reaches ketosis will depend on several factors, such as your metabolic resting rate, your body's fat percentage, and more.

Types of Keto Diets

The keto diet allows you to consume high-fat, low-carb foods. It also requires you to cut back on processed food items, sweets, starchy vegetables, and grains. If you're able to follow the diet well, you will be able to experience all the health benefits just like all the other individuals who have found success with this diet. The best thing about the keto diet is that there are a few types that you can choose from, including the following:

The Standard Ketogenic Diet, or SKD

The macronutrient ratio of this diet is 5–10 percent carbohydrates, 15–20 percent protein, and 75 percent fats. When you follow this diet, you need to plan all your snacks and meals around foods that are rich in fat. This is because you need to consume around 150 grams of fat each day so your body will start burning the fat for fuel. You also have to cut back on your carbohydrate intake, only eating 50 grams or less.

The Targeted Ketogenic Diet, or TKD

The macronutrient ratio of this diet is 10–15 percent carbohydrates, 20 percent protein, and 65–70 percent fat. This type of keto diet is very popular among active individuals, such as athletes. Unlike the standard keto diet, you're allowed to eat more carbohydrates right after or before working out.

The Cyclical Ketogenic Diet, or CKD

The macronutrient ratio of this diet is 5–10 percent carbohydrates, 15–20 percent protein, and 75 percent fat on "keto days." During "off days," the macronutrient ratio is 50 percent carbohydrates, 25 percent protein, and 25 percent fat. This type of keto diet allows you to cycle in and out of ketosis so that you can enjoy a balanced diet during your "off days."

The High-Protein Ketogenic Diet, or HPKD

The macronutrient ratio of this diet is 5–10 percent carbohydrates, 30 percent protein, and 60–65 percent fat. While following this type of keto diet, you should consume at least 120 grams of protein and 130 grams of fat each day. A lot of people prefer this diet because it allows them to consume less fat and more protein than the other types. However, following this diet might not allow you to achieve ketosis.

The Ketogenic Diet Basics

What is the Ketogenic Diet

The production of ketone bodies into the bloodstream will cause a situation called ketosis. Once the body has attained ketosis, most cells will use the ketone bodies to generate energy. The shift from using Carbohydrates to use of ketone bodies happens after 2 to 4 days of taking a diet that has 20 to 50 grams of carbohydrates. However, it is imperative to note that the process is based on an individual some people need more restriction to attain ketosis while others require a short time.

Since the diet lacks carbohydrates, the ketogenic diet is rich in fats and proteins. It includes meals with plenty of eggs, meats, cheeses, fish, butter, oils, and seeds as well as fibrous vegetables. The body likes to utilize glucose for energy however, this is not the most efficient source of energy because it brings serious health problems such as obesity, diabetes among other problems associated with a high carbohydrate diet. Glucose is the primary source of energy for your cells in the body, and when the levels of glucose are high, they are not burnt, and this, in turn, will result in the conversion of the glucose molecules to glycogen. Glycogen is stored in the peripheral and visceral organs leading to obesity.

However, as we age, we need foods that will give us adequate energy, and it is easily metabolized to reduce the chances of developing lifestyle diseases such as diabetes. The keto diet brings the body to ketosis the body will utilize the fats for energy.

Getting into Ketosis

When you are over 50, you will need to look at different changes that occur in the body. These changes will determine the quality of life that you will live in. Making dietary changes is an essential aspect that can go a long way in boosting your youthfulness. You will lose unwanted weight without the need to step into a gym. The keto diet has proven to be effective for people with a background of health issues such as obesity, blood sugar issues, and those who are suffering from emotional eating. Before we go into much details about the keto diet, we should get some background information about it.

The keto diet was developed in 1924 by Dr. Russel as a treatment of epileptic patients. However, over time, there are beneficial aspects of this diet that people are applying in their lives and enhancing their livelihood. He observed that when the body is in ketosis, it will prevent the onset of epileptic symptoms hence curing the condition. There are other benefits of the diet, which include: healing of brain injuries, preventing heart attack, maintaining a perfect level of blood glucose, treating autism, among others. a

Our bodies' functions and processes are different when you compare someone who is in their 20 or 30s versus an individual who is over 50 years. The main reason is that the level of metabolism tends to diminish over time, and you will need a diet that can cope up with the changes in your body. The keto diet is varied, and you can just adjust a few changes and enjoy all the meals that you want. It is important to note that it supports low carbs, and this is good because it helps in transitioning to a good healthy lifestyle. The younger generation is more robust and can handle quick changes, but over 50 individuals will take time to adjust to changes, especially dietary changes. You might experience headaches, nausea, fatigue, and dizziness. However, this is not the reason to quit you should look for focus and attention to help you achieve your target. You should not be worried or feel dejected because you are facing a myriad of challenges adapting to the diet.

When I am in Ketosis

Ketogenic Diets works by draining your body of the sugar that is in it, in order for the fat and protein to be isolated, causing ketosis (and weight loss).

1. Weight loss

A ketogenic diet can assist speed with increasing weight loss. Furthermore, since the diet is immense in energy, meaning it makes you less hungry than usual. In a meta-examination of 13 diverse experiments, five results uncovered huge weight loss from a keto diet.

2. Diminishes skin infections

There are many variables for skin break out, and one can be determined with diet and glucose. Eating a diet balancedprepared and refined starches can modify gut microscopic organisms and affects increasingly sensational glucose variances, in which two can have an impact on skin health. Therefore, by lessening carb admission, it is anything but expected that a keto diet could decrease a few instance of skin infections.

3. May secure mind working

More research is required into the keto diet and the mind. A few investigations propose that the ketogenic diet has neuroprotective benefits. Which is very helpful for treating or forestall conditions as Alzheimer Parkinson's, and even some rest issue. One investigation even found that youngsters following a ketogenic diet had improved sharpness and psychological working.

4. Possibly lessens seizures

It's the idea that the blend of fat, protein, and carbs modifies the manner in which the body utilizes vitality, bringing about ketosis. Ketosis is a raised degree of ketone bodies in the blood.

Ketosis can prompt a decrease in seizures in individuals with epilepsy.

5. Improves health in women with PCOS

Polycystic ovarian disorder (PCOS) is an endocrine issue that causes augmented ovaries with pimples. A high-sugar diet can contrarily influence those with PCOS.

There aren't numerous clinical examinations on the ketogenic diet and PCOS. One pilot study that included five women over a 24-week time frame found that the ketogenic diet:

- *increased weight loss*
- *aided hormone balance*
- *improved luteinizing hormone (LH)/follicle-invigorating hormone (FSH) proportions*
- improved fasting insulin

Keto is often recommended for kids who experience the ill effects of the specific issue (like Lennox-Gastaut disorder or Rett disorder) and don't react to seizure prescription, as indicated by the Epilepsy Foundation.

Benefits of Ketogenic Diet

If you're a person who's already celebrated your 50th birthday, that doesn't mean that your life becomes dull from here on, and you don't know how to spend your free time. Quite the opposite! You may often feel time-crunch because of work, family, and generally because of various life situations. Actually, it can be quite difficult to make time for yourself and, moreover, finding time to plan a healthy diet is more likely to be last on the list of your priorities. However, you can change your attitude towards your nutritional needs and move them to the top of that list when you find out all the benefits of a low-carb, high-fat diet for older people.

Improved Physical and Mental Health

With ageing you might notice an energy level drop due to different environmental and biological reasons. If you want to feel happy, active, and dynamic, pay closer attention to the Keto diet. Remember, reducing your carbohydrate intake usually leads to increasing your vital forces. When you start consuming a lower number of carbs, the body has to burn more fat to fuel itself. This process causes fat synthesis and ketone production, i.e. breaking down accumulated fat for energy. In such a way, the low-carbohydrate diet can stimulate brainpower and positive changes in cognition (like improving memory and concentration).

Faster Metabolism

Older people have a slower metabolism. But thanks to the Keto diet, this problem can be solved. Excluding carb intake from your diet plan can help you to maintain healthy levels of blood sugar and, as a result, rev up your metabolism.

Weight-Shedding

It is no big secret that as a person gets older, shedding weight gets harder. People after 50 face the challenge of weight-loss for a variety of reasons (from increasing levels of stress, slower metabolic rate to rapid muscle loss). The struggle with excess weight may take a lot of time and effort for people over the age of 50. But there is a way out, and it is called the Keto diet.

This peculiar diet is highly effective for losing weight because it boosts the metabolism of fat, and the body itself starts shedding stored fat. As an added bonus, people who stick to the Keto diet get a reduced appetite, which helps to prevent over-eating and, thus, quicker weight loss. Unlike many low-fat diets, the Ketogenic one doesn't recommend you to track your calories or eat less. There's no need for that! Keto usually leaves you feeling full and satisfied after a meal.

Better Sleep

At an old age, people tend to have trouble sleeping. A lot of people over 50 experience such sleep disorders as insomnia, sleep apnea, restless leg syndrome, and sleepwalking. People aged 50 and over should know that a long-term Ketogenic diet can have a positive impact on sleep. A significant reduction in carb intake and, at the same time, a substantial increase in fat intake create favorable conditions for a night of deeper sleep, eliminate certain sleep disturbance triggers, and make a person more energetic when the sun is up.

Protection from Age-Related Diseases

According to various scientific studies, the Keto diet can reduce the risks for specific age-related diseases, such as diabetes, different kinds of cancer, cardiovascular diseases, mental disorders, Parkinson's Disease, multiple sclerosis, and fatty liver disease.

Keto Diet FAQs

Why are you here?

OK – first things first – why are you here? Do you want to lose weight or do you want to just have a healthier lifestyle?

Following this dietary plan will give you all three of these results – but finding out your ultimate goal will help you better plan your diet to achieve those goals. For example, if you're already happy with your weight and only want to have a healthier lifestyle, then you don't have to adhere so strictly to the carbohydrate requirement.

This is why I always encourage going to your primary physician first to find out what your dietary limits are. This was the first mistake I made when I decided to follow a weight loss regiment. Keep in mind – we're trying to improve the quality of your life and not make it worse.

Is there such a thing as too much fat?

Everything in moderation. If you consume too much of one thing, it doesn't matter even if its water – it will be too bad for you. So yes, you can eat too much fat. Remember how we talked about the importance of calories? Well, you have to understand that of all the nutrients found today, fat is perhaps the most compact type. This means that each gram of fat has more calories than any other nutrients you can find today.

What does this mean? This means that if you eat too much fat, there's a good chance that you'll go beyond your calorie requirements. If your goal is weight loss or maintaining a healthy weight, then this is a bad route to take because you won't be experiencing a calorie deficit. Simply put – you'd actually gain weight instead of losing it. I want you to understand this because I don't want you eating more than you should in the mistaken belief that its "healthy" for you.

How much weight can you lose?

The amount of weight you can lose on the Ketogenic Diet depends primarily on how well you stick to the plan. The healthy rate is 2 pounds per week and I strongly recommend that you don't speed it up too much. As mentioned, I lost 30 pounds on the diet – but this took years of hard work and personal research on my part!

Should I be counting calories?

Generally, counting calories is the go-to for people who want to lose weight. You will find however that this is not a problem when you're on a Keto Diet. That doesn't mean you should forget calories altogether – it only means that it's not that big of an issue in the grand scheme of things.

So the question is – how many calories should you be eating if you're on a Ketogenic Diet? Well, this depends from one person to the next. You will find that there are calculators that can help you get the proper amount of calories you want to maintain while on Keto. A good online calculator is known as the Mifflin St. Jeor calculator which allows for a calorie suggestion based on your height, weight, and age.

Of course, if you want to be challenged, here's the typical formula.

For males: 10 multiplied by weight in kilograms + 6.25 x height in centimeters less 5 multiplied by age + 5

For females: 10 multiplied by weight in kilograms + 6.25 x height in centimeters less 5 multiplied by age – 161

Once you get the results, you'll have to multiply it using the following situations:

- Sedentary: x 1.2, if you have minimal physical activities such as having a desk job

- Lightly active: x 1.375 light jogging at least once a week

- Moderately active: x 1.55 moderate activity, at least 6 times a week

- Very active: x 1.725 hard exercise daily or hard exercise twice a week

So it's a little tough – but the online calculator should make the whole thing easier. Generally however, you'd want to maintain a calorie count of 1500 calories per day for weight loss. For health maintenance without the need to lose weight, you can hit 1800 to 2000 calories – depending on the level of activity you experience every day.

Here's the most important question however: do you have to be strict about it? The short answer is: YES. Just because you're on the Ketogenic Diet doesn't mean you can eat all the meat you want. This is not a free pass – you still have to be mindful of what you eat.

The good news is that if you follow the Ketogenic Diet strictly, you'll find that the period of satiation is longer. Simply put, you won't feel hungry so quickly on the diet. There will be no mid-afternoon cravings for a snack as you feel full all through the hours between lunch and dinner. Even if you *do* feel hungry, there are a bunch of Keto-friendly snacks you can reach for.

Keto Grocery List

I've had people complain about the difficulty of switching their grocery list to one that's Ketogenic-friendly. The fact is that food is expensive – and most of the food you have in your fridge are probably packed full with carbohydrates. This is why if you're committing to a Ketogenic Diet, you need to do a clean sweep. That's right – everything that's packed with carbohydrates should be identified and set aside to make sure you're not eating more than you should. You can donate them to a charity before going out and buying your new Keto-friendly shopping list.

- Seafood
- Low-carb Vegetables
- Fruits Low in Sugar
- Meat and Eggs
- Nuts and Seeds

- Dairy Products
- Oils
- Coffee and Tea
- Dark Chocolate
- Sugar Substitutes

Ketogenic Diet for Men and Women Over 50

The relationship between Aging and Nutritional Need

As we age, you can expect a number of different changes to happen in your body, including thinner skin, loss of muscle, and less stomach acid. When these things happen, this can, unfortunately, make you more prone to nutrient deficiencies and overall quality of life. This is where the Ketogenic Diet comes in handy! By eating a variety of foods and incorporating the proper supplements, you will be able to meet your nutrient needs with no issues! Below, you will find some of the effects of aging and how to help the issue.

Less Calories- More Nutrients

On a general basis, an individual's daily calorie count will depend on a number of factors, including activity level, muscle mass, weight, and height. As for us older adults, we will need to begin lowering the number of calories we take in, in order to maintain or lose weight. Generally, older adults tend to exercise and move less compared to younger individuals.

While consuming fewer calories, it is important to continue getting higher levels of nutrients. For this reason, it is highly suggested to consume a variety of foods such as low-carb vegetables and lean meats to help get the proper nutrients and fight against any nutrient deficiencies. The nutrients you will want to focus on include vitamin B12, calcium, and vitamin D, Magnesium, Potassium, Omega-3 fatty acids, and Iron.

Benefits of Fiber

While many people do not like to discuss this, constipation is a prevalent health issue for individuals over the age of 50. In fact, women over the age of 65 are two to three times more likely to experience constipation! This may be due to the fact that people over the age of 50 generally move less and are more likely to be taking a medication that has constipation as an unfortunate side effect.

To help relieve constipation, you will want to make sure you are getting enough fiber. When you eat more fiber, it is able to pass through your gut, undigested, and help regulate bowel movements and form stool. As an added benefit, high-fiber diets may also be able to prevent diverticular disease. Diverticular disease is a condition where small pouches build along the wall of the colon and become inflamed.

Focus on Protein

It will be essential to find a balance on your new diet. As we age, it is very common to lose both strength and muscle. In fact, on average, an adult will lose anywhere between 3-8% of their muscle mass per decade after the age of 30. When we lose muscle mass, it could lead to poor health, fractures, and weakness among an elderly population. By eating more protein, you can help fight sarcopenia and maintain your muscle mass.

Vitamin B12

As mentioned earlier, keeping up with proper nutrients is going to be vital for your health. One of the vitamins you will want to focus on is Vitamin B12. This is a water-soluble vitamin that is in charge of making red blood cells and keeping your brain healthy. Unfortunately, it is estimated that anywhere from 1—30% of individuals over the age of 50 have a lowered ability to absorb this vitamin from their diet.

One of the main reasons individuals over the age of 50 have difficulty absorbing vitamin B12 may be due to the fact that they have reduced stomach acid reduction. Vitamin B12 is bound to proteins. In order for your body to use this vitamin, the stomach acid separates it from the protein and becomes absorbed. To benefit your new diet, you will want to consider taking a supplement of vitamin B12 or consuming foods that are fortified with the vitamin.

Vitamin D and Calcium

When it comes to bone health, calcium and vitamin D are going to be very important. While calcium is in charge of maintaining and building healthy bones, it depends on vitamin D to help the body absorb the calcium in the first place! Unfortunately, adults have a harder time absorbing calcium in their diets. This may be due to the fact that the gut absorbs less calcium as we age. However, the main culprit of a reduction in calcium is typically due to a vitamin D deficiency. As you can tell, they work hand in hand!

The reason we may experience a vitamin D deficiency is due to thinning skin. Generally, our body makes vitamin D from the cholesterol in the skin when it is exposed to sunlight. As the skin becomes thinner, it reduces the ability to make vitamin D and, in turn, reduces the ability to get enough calcium. When these two things happen, it increases the risk of fractures and bone loss.

To help counter this aging effect, you will want to make sure you are getting enough vitamin D and calcium in your diet. Some accessible sources will be dairy products, leafy vegetables, and dark greens. As far as Vitamin D goes, you will want to include a variety of fish or even a Vitamin D supplement such as cod liver oil.

Dehydration

On the Ketogenic Diet or not, staying hydrated is important at any age. In fact, water makes up about 60% of our bodies! Whether you are 20,30, or 50, the body still continually loses water through urine and sweat. As we age, it makes us more prone to dehydration.

When we become dehydrated, the water detects the thirst through receptors found all throughout the body and the brain. As we age, the receptors become less sensitive, making it hard to distinguish the thirst in the first place. On top of this, our kidneys are there to help converse water, but they also lose function with age.

Unfortunately, the consequences of dehydration are pretty harsh for the older population. When you are dehydrated long-term, this could reduce your ability to absorb medication and could worsen any medical condition. For this reason, it will be vital you keep up with your intake of water. I suggest trying a water challenge with friends and family or try having a glass of water with each meal you have.

Appetite

One of the last topics we will tackle on the subject of aging it the decrease in appetite. While this may seem like a benefit, a lack of eating could lead to a number of different nutritional deficiencies and unwanted weight loss. Poor appetite is most commonly linked to a heightened risk of death and overall poor health.

It is believed that some of the significant factors behind appetite loss could be due to changes in smell, taste, and hormones. Generally, older adults who have lower levels of hunger have higher levels of fullness hormones. When this happens, it causes individuals to be less hungry overall. As we age, the changes in smell and taste can also make food seem less appealing.

If you find this happens to you, you may want to establish a healthy habit of snacking. When you snack, try to reach for keto-friendly foods such as eggs, yogurt, and almonds to help put the nutrients back into your diet. If you are aware of this issue, it is something you can get a grasp on before it becomes a real problem.

How Proper Nutrition Helps Slow Down Aging

Some products are promoted as ways to slow or prevent the aging process. However, none of them is as effective as choosing the right diet. One of the main aspects that you should consider is the diet. Proper nutrition is essential in slowing down the aging process naturally because you will be replenishing your brain and body cells as well. Some of the factors that you should look into include:

a) Calories

As we age, the resting metabolic rate will decline. This is one area that will lead to undesirable weight gain, and this can increase the chances of getting specific chronic diseases. The decrease in metabolic rate is related to the loss of lean body mass. The way you can avoid this is by following a healthy diet and increase your physical activity to help in strengthening your muscles and raise your metabolic rate.

b) Proteins

Proteins are a vital component in cellular growth, repair, and maintenance. Despite the need to consume lower calories, you should ensure that your nutrition has adequate proteins.

c) Dental Health

It is estimated that over 81% of the adult population has periodontal disease. You must observe nutrition that will boost teeth maintenance or foods with fluoride. You should incorporate more fruits and vegetables. You should have all your teeth to enjoy your meals, and this is where you should focus on maintaining good oral care.

d) Taste

The taste and smell are dulled by the aging process. However, you can revamp it by staying hydrated throughout and resisting the use of salt shaker. You can use herbs to enhance flavor in foods.

e) Antioxidants

Antioxidants are essential nutritional components that slow down the aging process. The antioxidants can help in preventing chronic diseases and slow down the aging process.

f) Calcium And Vitamin d

The majority of the body requires calcium ions and vitamin D as we age. The mineral is essential for the proper functioning of the nervous system, blood clotting, and muscle contractions. Adequate calcium intake is essential in slowing down the aging process. In addition to the nutrients, you should always take an adequate amount of water to prevent dehydration and loss of vital chemicals.

How Calories Restriction Slows Down Aging

For anyone who has never tracked their calories and learned the quality ratio of protein, fat, and carbohydrates that is effective for their body. When you monitor your calories for a few days, you will know what your body needs and what you can do to enhance your health. You need a diet that will give you adequate energy throughout the day and boost cellular regeneration. There are reasons why the restriction of calories will slow down the aging process. Some of the benefits of calorie restriction include:

Flexibility And Customization

There is no one size fits all macros because everyone has their health objectives. However, when you choose the best calorie intake that will put your health goals forward, you will be able to make the right decision and reduce the cellular aging process. It is important to understand that cells age when they are not rejuvenated properly. When you restrict calories and choose one which improves cellular division, you will remain youthful.

You Will Have More Balance In Your Diet

Unlike other restrictive diets, you can monitor your calories and still enjoy the foods that you love. A ketogenic diet will reduce fat deposits in the peripheral and visceral organs, which often causes obesity, among other conditions. When your macronutrients are balanced, you will always feel energized and rejuvenated.

Easily manage medical conditions

Some studies indicate that managing your calorie intake is essential in building a better feeling and rejuvenation. Studies indicate that the macronutrients will help you manage conditions such as diabetes, polycystic ovary syndrome, and certain cancers. You must consult your physician before cutting down your calories.

Tips and Tricks to be Learnt about Keto Diet For Seniors

I guess I have been able to establish the fact that as a senior, you can't do Keto as everyone else will. This is right because you have specific needs to milk off the lifestyle.

Working around your Keto diet, and suiting it to the nutritional needs of the body is vital. Below, I'll be listing some changes and twists that can be made to the diet. This is to maintain immune function, prevent bone and muscle loss, preserve eyesight, and protect cells from damage.

- Eat more veggies, fruits, whole grains, fish, beans, and low-fat or fat-free dairyand keep meat and poultry lean.

- Drink plenty of water

- Change your eating pattern, now, eat small meals rather than huge sized meals, but make sure to eat more often.

- Trying doing more of strength training

- Take more calcium-laden meals

Getting Your Calories Right

While on Keto, you do not necessarily have to track every calorie intake. There is a general macronutrient breakdown that you can follow to track your intake. Although, like I already established, the macro ratio- 60-80% fats, 5% carbs, and 35-15% protein, is a broad estimate and is not particular to your needs. So you should calculate your macro count for your self.

To effectively track your macros, know and adhere strictly to your macro counts, invest in a food scale, and know what you eat.

Learn to Track Your Ketosis

There is no standard duration of time for which anyone can enter Ketosis, for some people, it is, in fact, a tug of war. It is only reasonable that some people get into Ketosis earlier than others. So have it at the back of your mind that the time taken to enter Ketosis varies from person to person. One major factor is your rate of carb intake before the commencement of your Keto journey. If you used to take carbs in large quantities before you began the Keto plan, then it will take a longer period for your body to burn up all the stored glycogen. And then, begin to produce Ketones.

But on a very broadly general note, it takes 2 to 4 days to reach Ketosis if you eat about 50 grams of carbs per day, however, do not take this as the standard. Factors that can, however, help you speed up the pace of your intake of carbs, daily consumption of fats, and protein and your rate of metabolism.

To track your Ketosis, you should consistently measure your Ketone levels. You can check it with a breath meter, a urine strip, or a blood ketone meter. These tools measure acetone, acetoacetate, and beta-hydroxybutyrate, respectively.

It is essential because it is possible to fall out of the metabolic state.

How to Keep Your Ketosis Running

To be able to get the best out of Keto, your body must necessarily enter Ketosis. And it doesn't just end there your body does not only have to enter Ketosis but must maintain the Ketosis state. And to achieve this, much planning has to go into your dieting. Below are some tips that can ensure that you maintain Ketosis.

Track your carb intake. Ensure that you are eating 20-50 grams of carbs daily. Do not consume more or less than the required carb intake, as suggested in your macro reading.

Watch out for hidden carb sources. Like salad dressings, sauces, and all. It would help if you regulated the rate at which you eat out. Bring it to the barest minimum.

Exercise regularly, it can help empty carb stores, for those who are probably unintentionally taking more carbs than they should.

Consider intermittent fasting. Although this is more useful for people that are trying to get into Ketosis, it still applies to maintaining Ketosis.

Test your Ketone levels regularly. It is the most important tip. Because this is what will tell you the further step to take note that just like overloading your body with carbs can disrupt the Ketosis process, underestimating your carb count can be bad for your body too.

A blood Ketone level of 1.5-3.0 mmol per liter is okay to keep your Ketosis running.

Tips on Maintaining Ketosis For Senior Over 50

Find Your Macros

This is one of the most important aspects of maintaining ketosis in your system. You should know the macronutrients that you require and what are your health objectives. When you know this, you can make the right decision. You can experiment on the levels until you get a level that your body can cope up with, and you are comfortable. The standard ketogenic diet falls around 35% protein, 5% carbs, and 60% fats.

Track Your Carbs To Stay Ketotic

One of the main aspects that will help you in maintaining ketosis is by tracking your carbohydrate levels. The carbs intake should be kept very low and fats so high to help the body to utilize the fats for energy. You will not attain ketosis if you maintain a high level of carbohydrates.

Test Your Ketone Levels

One of the main benefits of ketosis is that you do not just follow the diet. You can also measure the levels of ketone bodies in the system. You can know the right amount of proteins and fats in your body to help you maintain the state. You will be able to know if your body is generating adequate ketones.

Food to Avoid

It is important to note that asides from the long list of food that you should avoid while on a keto diet, there are some foods that you have to keep away. It is true as a result of the age factor. Primary among the foods to stay away from are:

- Peanuts
- Lentils
- Sugars and sweeteners

- Beans
- Rice
- Pasta
- Oatmeal
- Low-fat dairy products
- Corn
- Starchy vegetable
- Soda
- Potatoes
- Wine (excess consumption)

30-Day Meal Plan For People Over 50

Okay, so you we're given recipes above to help start your journey towards a Keto-friendly diet. I understand however that many of those recipes are a bit more complicated than most – especially if you're a complete beginner. Chances are you're having a hard time with the groceries and the unknown food items that are suddenly included in your grocery list.

While you're strongly encouraged to do some shopping and try out many of the recipes I gave above, I understand how this healthier lifestyle is a bit new to you.

30-Day Meal Plan Sample

Day	Breakfast	Lunch	Dinner
1	Almond Coconut Egg Wraps	Super Salmon Parcel	Winter Comfort stew
2	Bacon & Avocado Omelet	New England Salmon Pie	Ideal Cold Weather Stew
3	Bacon & Cheese Frittata	Juicy Garlic Butter Shrimp	Weekend Dinner Stew
4	Bacon & Egg Breakfast Muffins	Simple Lemon Garlic Shrimp	Mexican Pork Stew
5	Bacon Hash	Flavorful Shrimp Creole	Hungarian Pork Stew
6	Bagels With Cheese	Creamy Scallops	Yellow Chicken Soup
7	Baked Apples	Perfect Pan-Seared Scallops	Curry Soup

8	Baked Eggs In The Avocado	Easy Baked Shrimp Scampi	Delicious Tomato Basil Soup
9	Banana Pancakes	Delicious Blackened Shrimp	Chicken Enchilada Soup
10	Breakfast Skillet	Creamy Parmesan Shrimp	Buffalo Chicken Soup
11	Brunch BLT Wrap	Pan Fry Shrimp & Zucchini	Slow Cooker Taco Soup
12	Cheesy Bacon & Egg Cups	Chicken avocado salad	Wedding Soup
13	Coconut Keto Porridge	Low carb Caesar salad	Slow Cooker Taco Soup
14	Cream Cheese Eggs	Keto broccoli salad	Classic Pork Tenderloin
15	Creamy Basil Baked Sausage	Keto chicken-cheese salad	Signature Italian Pork Dish
16	Holiday Morning Bread	Keto hamburger salad	Flavor Packed Pork Loin
17	Masterpiece Bread	Keto tomato and avocado salad	Spiced Pork Tenderloin
18	Dense Morning Bread	Calamari mayo with cauliflower broccoli salad	Sticky Pork Ribs
19	Multi Seeds Bread	Chicken Spinach salad	Valentine's Day Dinner

20	Sandwich Bread	Eggplant Lasagna	South East Asian Steak Platter
21	Magic Cheese Bread	Keto Vegan Cauliflower and Tofu Stir Fry	Pesto Flavored Steak
22	10-Minutes Bread	Keto Vegan Curry	Flawless Grilled Steak
23	Subtle Rosemary Bread	Shirataki Noodles With Vegan Alfredo Sauce	Mongolian Beef
24	Brunch Time Bread	Slow Cooker Taco Soup	Sicilian Steak Pinwheel
25	Amazing Cheddar Bread	Wedding Soup	American Beef Wellington
26	Grain-Free Creamy Noodles	Slow Cooker Taco Soup	Pastry-Free Beef Wellington
27	Meat-Free Zoodles Stroganoff	Classic Pork Tenderloin	Eggplant Lasagna
28	Eye-Catching Veggies	Signature Italian Pork Dish	Keto Vegan Cauliflower and Tofu Stir Fry
29	Favorite Punjabi Curry	Sticky Pork Ribs	Keto broccoli salad
30	Traditional Indian Curry	Valentine's Day Dinner	Pan Fry Shrimp & Zucchini

Keto Breakfast Recipes

1. Almond Coconut Egg Wraps

Preparation Time: 5 minutes

Cooking Time: 5 minutes

Servings: 4

Ingredients:

Organic eggs (5)

Coconut flour (1 tbsp.)

Sea salt (.25 tsp.)

Almond meal (2 tbsp.)

Directions:

Combine the fixings in a blender and work them until creamy. Heat a skillet using the med-high temperature setting.

Pour two tablespoons of batter into the skillet and cook - covered about three minutes. Turn it over to cook for another 3 minutes. Serve the wraps piping hot.

Nutrition:

Carbohydrates: 3 grams

Protein: 8 grams

Fats: 8 grams

Calories: 111

2. Bacon & Avocado Omelet

Preparation Time: 5 minutes

Cooking Time: 5 minutes

Servings: 1

Ingredients:

Crispy bacon (1 slice)

Large organic eggs (2)

Freshly grated parmesan cheese (.5 cup)

Ghee or coconut oil or butter (2 tbsp.)

Avocado (half of 1 small)

Directions:

Prepare the bacon to your liking and set aside. Combine the eggs, parmesan cheese, and your choice of finely chopped herbs. Warm a skillet and add the butter/ghee to melt using the medium-high heat setting. When the pan is hot, whisk and add the eggs.

Prepare the omelet working it towards the middle of the pan for about 30 seconds. When firm, flip, and cook it for another 30 seconds. Arrange the omelet on a plate and garnish with the crunched bacon bits. Serve with sliced avocado.

Nutrition:

Carbohydrates: 3.3 grams

Protein: 30 grams

Fats: 63 grams

Calories: 719

3. Bacon & Cheese Frittata

Preparation Time: 5 minutes

Cooking Time: 5 minutes

Servings: 6

Ingredients:

Heavy cream (1 cup)   Eggs (6)

Crispy slices of bacon (5)

Chopped green onions (2)

Cheddar cheese (4 oz.)

Also Needed: 1 pie plate

Directions:

Warm the oven temperature to reach 350° Fahrenheit.

Whisk the eggs and seasonings. Empty into the pie pan and top off with the remainder of the fixings. Bake 30-35 minutes. Wait for a few minutes before serving for the best results.

Nutrition: Protein: 13 grams

Carbohydrates: 2 grams

Fats: 29 grams

Calories: 320

4. Bacon & Egg Breakfast Muffins

Preparation Time: 15 minutes

Cooking Time: 30 minutes

Servings: 12

Ingredients:

Eggs (8 large)

Bacon (8 slices)

Green onion (.66 cup)

Directions:

Warm the oven at 350° Fahrenheit. Spritz the muffin tin wells using a cooking oil spray. Chop the onions and set aside.

Prepare a large skillet using the medium temperature setting. Fry the bacon until it's crispy and place on a layer of paper towels to drain the grease. Chop it into small pieces after it has cooled.

Whisk the eggs, bacon, and green onions, mixing well until all of the fixings are incorporated. Dump the egg mixture into the muffin tin (halfway full). Bake it for about 20 to 25 minutes. Cool slightly and serve.

Nutrition:

Carbohydrates: 0.4 grams

Protein: 5.6 grams

Fats: 4.9 grams

Calories: 69

5. Bacon Hash

Preparation Time: 5 minutes

Cooking Time: 10 minutes

Servings: 2

Ingredients:

Small green pepper (1)

Jalapenos (2)

Small onion (1)

Eggs (4)

Bacon slices (6)

Directions:

Chop the bacon into chunks using a food processor. Set aside for now. Slice the onions and peppers into thin strips.

Dice the jalapenos as small as possible.

Heat a skillet and fry the veggies. Once browned, combine the fixings and cook until crispy. Place on a serving dish with the eggs.

Nutrition:

Carbohydrates: 9 grams

Protein: 23 grams

Fats: 24 grams

Calories: 366

6. Bagels With Cheese

Preparation Time: 10 minutes

Cooking Time: 15 minutes

Servings: 6

Ingredients:

Mozzarella cheese (2.5 cups)

Baking powder (1 tsp.)

Cream cheese (3 oz.)

Almond flour (1.5 cups)

Eggs (2)

Directions:

Shred the mozzarella and combine with the flour, baking powder, and cream cheese in a mixing container. Pop into the microwave for about one minute. Mix well.

Let the mixture cool and add the eggs. Break apart into six sections and shape into round bagels. *Note*: You can also sprinkle with a seasoning of your choice or pinch of salt if desired.

Bake them for approximately 12 to 15 minutes. Serve or cool and store.

Nutrition:

Carbohydrates: 8 grams

Protein: 19 grams

Fats: 31 grams

Calories: 374

7. Baked Apples

Preparation Time: 10 minutes

Cooking Time: 1 hour

Servings: 4

Ingredients:

Keto-friendly sweetener (4 tsp. or to taste)

Cinnamon (.75 tsp.)

Chopped pecans (.25 cup)

Granny Smith apples (4 large)

Directions:

Set the oven temperature at 375° Fahrenheit. Mix the sweetener with the cinnamon and pecans. Core the apple and add the prepared stuffing.

Add enough water into the baking dish to cover the bottom of the apple. Bake them for about 45 minutes to 1 hour.

Nutrition:

Carbohydrates: 16 grams

Protein: 6.8 grams

Fats: 19.9 grams

Calories: 175

8. Baked Eggs In The Avocado

Preparation Time: 10 minutes

Cooking Time: 20 minutes

Servings: 1

Ingredients:

Avocado (half of 1)

Egg (1)   Olive oil (1 tbsp.)

Shredded cheddar cheese (.5 cup)

Directions:

Heat the oven to reach 425° Fahrenheit.

Discard the avocado pit and remove just enough of the 'insides' to add the egg. Drizzle with oil and break the egg into the shell.

Sprinkle with cheese and bake them for 15 to 16 minutes until the egg is the way you prefer. Serve.

Nutrition: Fats: 52 grams

Carbohydrates: 3 grams

Protein: 21 grams

Calories: 452

9. Banana Pancakes

Preparation Time: 10 minutes

Cooking Time: 15 minutes

Servings: 3

Ingredients:

Butter (as needed)

Bananas (2) Eggs (4)

Cinnamon (1 tsp.)

Optional: Baking powder (.5 tsp.)

Directions:

Combine each of the fixings. Melt a portion of butter in a skillet using the medium temperature setting. Prepare the pancakes 1-2 minutes per side. Cook them with the lid on for the first part of the cooking cycle for a fluffier pancake. Serve plain or with your favorite garnishes such as a dollop of coconut cream or fresh berries.

Nutrition:

Carbohydrates: 6.8 grams

Fats: 7 grams

Calories: 157

10. Breakfast Skillet

Preparation Time: 10 minutes | **Cooking Time:** 15 minutes | **Servings:** 2

Ingredients:

Organic ground turkey/grass-fed beef (.75-1 lb.)

Organic eggs (6)

Keto-friendly salsa of choice (1 cup)

Directions: Warm the skillet using oil (medium heat). Add the turkey and simmer until the pink is gone. Fold in the salsa and simmer for two to three minutes. Crack the eggs and add to the top of the turkey base. Place a lid on the pot and cook for seven minutes until the whites of the eggs are opaque.

Note: The **Cooking Time** will vary depending on how you like the eggs prepared

Nutrition:

Carbohydrates: 7.1 grams

Protein: 65.2 grams

Fats: 32 grams

Calories: 556

11. Brunch BLT Wrap

Preparation Time: 5 minutes

Cooking Time: 15 minutes

Servings: 1

Ingredients:

Crispy fried bacon slices (4)

Romaine or Iceberg lettuce leaves (2)

Chopped tomatoes (.25 cup)

Mayo (1 tbsp.)

Optional: Pepper

Directions:

Cook the bacon until crispy in a skillet or the microwave (your choice). Spread a layer of mayonnaise on one side of the lettuce.

Add the bacon and tomato. Season the wrap to your liking. Roll it up and serve.

Nutrition:

Carbohydrates: 2 grams

Protein: 8 grams

Fats: 24 grams

Calories: 256

12. Cheesy Bacon & Egg Cups

Preparation Time: 10 minutes

Cooking Time: 20 minutes

Servings: 6

Ingredients:

Bacon (6 strips)

Large eggs (6)

Cheese (.25 cup)

Fresh spinach (1 handful)

Pepper (as desired)

Directions:

Set the oven setting to 400° Fahrenheit.

Prepare the bacon using medium heat on the stovetop. Place it on towels to drain.

Grease six muffin tins with a spritz of oil. Line each tin with a slice of bacon, pressing tightly to make a secure well for the eggs.

Drain and dry the spinach with a paper towel. Whisk the eggs and combine with the spinach.

Add the mixture to the prepared tins and sprinkle with cheese. Sprinkle with salt and pepper until it's like you like it.

Bake for 15 minutes. Remove when done and serve or cool to store in the fridge.

Nutrition:

Carbohydrates: 1 gram

Protein: 8 grams

Fats: 7 grams

Calories: 101

13. Coconut Keto Porridge

Preparation Time: 15 minutes

Cooking Time: 10 minutes

Servings: 1

Ingredients:

Coconut cream (4 tbsp.)

Ground psyllium husk powder (1 pinch)

Coconut flour (1 tbsp.)

Flaxseed egg (1)

Coconut butter (1 oz.)

Directions:

Toss all of the fixings together in a small pan before placing the pan on the stovetop burner set to low heat. Stir the mixture as it cooks to encourage the porridge to thicken. Continue stirring until your preferred thickness is reached.

A small amount of coconut milk or a few berries (fresh or frozen) can also be added to taste if desired.

Nutrition:

Carbohydrates: 5.4 grams

Protein: 10.1 grams

Fats: 22.8 grams

Calories: 401

14. Cream Cheese Eggs

Preparation Time: 5 minutes

Cooking Time: 5 minutes

Servings: 1

Ingredients:

Butter (1 tbsp.)

Eggs (2)

Soft cream cheese with chives (2 tbsp.)

Directions:

Preheat a skillet and melt the butter.

Whisk the eggs with the cream cheese.

Add to the pan and stir until done.

Nutrition:

Carbohydrates: 3 grams

Protein: 15 grams

Fats: 31 grams

Calories: 341

15. Creamy Basil Baked Sausage

Preparation Time: 5 minutes

Cooking Time: 5 minutes

Servings: 12

Ingredients:

Italian sausage - pork/turkey or chicken (3 lb.)

Cream cheese (8 oz.)

Heavy cream (.25 cup)

Basil pesto (.25 cup)

Mozzarella (8 oz.)

Directions:

Set the oven at 400° Fahrenheit.

Lightly spritz a casserole dish with cooking oil spray. Add the sausage to the dish and bake for 30 minutes. Combine the heavy cream, pesto, and cream cheese.

Pour the sauce over the casserole and top it off with the cheese.

Bake for another 10 minutes. The sausage should reach 160° Fahrenheit in the center when checked with a meat thermometer. You can also broil for 3 minutes to brown the cheesy layer.

Nutrition:

Carbohydrates: 4 grams

Protein: 23 grams

Fats: 23 grams

Calories: 316

Keto Bread Recipes

16. Holiday Morning Bread

Preparation Time: 15 minutes

Cooking Time: 50 minutes

Servings: 10

Ingredients:

1/3 C. unsweetened almond milk

¼ C. granulated Erythritol

2 tbsp. ground flax seeds

1 tsp. organic vanilla extract

¾ C. homemade pumpkin puree

½ C. coconut oil, softened

¾ C. organic soy flour

¼ C. coconut flour

½ tsp. organic baking powder

¼ tsp. baking soda

1 tsp. ground cinnamon

½ tsp. ground ginger

½ tsp. ground cardamom

¼ tsp. salt

Direction:

Preheat the oven to 3500 F. Line a 9x5-inch loaf pan with parchment paper.

In a bowl, add the almond milk, Erythritol, flax seeds and vanilla extract and mix until well combined.

Set aside for about 5 minutes.

Meanwhile, in another bowl, add the flours, baking powder, baking soda, spices and salt and mix until well combined.

In the bowl of almond milk, add the pumpkin puree and coconut oil and beat until well combined.

Add the flour mixture and mix until well combined and smooth.

Place the mixture into the prepared loaf pan evenly.

Bake for about 50 minutes or until a toothpick inserted in the center comes out clean.

Remove the bread pan from oven and place onto a wire rack to cool for about 10 minutes.

Carefully, invert the bread onto the wire rack to cool completely before slicing.

With a sharp knife, cut the bread loaf into the desired sized slices and serve.

Nutrition:

Calories: 150
Carbohydrates: 6.8g
Protein: 4.2g
Fat: 12.5g
Sugar: 2.2g
Sodium: 106mg
Fiber: 3g

17. Masterpiece Bread

Preparation Time: 15 minutes

Cooking Time: 45 minutes

Servings: 12

Ingredients:

8 large organic eggs, room temperature

¾ C. coconut flour

1/3 C. butter, melted

1 tsp. organic baking powder

1 tsp. organic vanilla extract

¼ tsp. salt

1/3 C. fresh raspberries

Direction:

Preheat the oven to 3500 F. Line a 9x5-inch loaf pan with parchment paper.

In a food processor, add the eggs and pulse on high speed until frothy and smooth.

Add the remaining ingredients except raspberries and pulse on high speed until smooth.

Place the mixture into the prepared loaf pan evenly.

Place the raspberries on top and gently, submerge into the dough.

Bake for about 40-45 minutes or until a toothpick inserted in the center comes out clean.

Remove the bread pan from oven and place onto a wire rack to cool for about 10 minutes.

Carefully, invert the bread onto the wire rack to cool completely before slicing.

With a sharp knife, cut the bread loaf into the desired sized slices and serve.

Nutrition:

Calories: 103
Carbohydrates: 1.9g
Protein: 4.4g
Fat: 8.6g
Sugar: 0.6g
Sodium: 233mg
Fiber: 0.6g

18. Dense Morning Bread

Preparation Time: 15 minutes

Cooking Time: 1 hour 10 minutes

Servings: 16

Ingredients:

2 C. blanched almond flour

2 tsp. organic baking powder

¼ tsp. salt

¾ C. Erythritol

½ C. butter, softened

3 large organic eggs

1 tbsp. fresh lemon juice

1 tbsp. fresh lemon zest, grated

1 tsp. organic vanilla extract

1½ C. zucchini, grated and squeezed

1 C. fresh blueberries

Direction:

Preheat the oven to 3250 F. Line a 9x5-inch loaf pan with parchment paper.

In a bowl, mix together the almond flour, baking powder and salt.

In another large bowl, add the Erythritol and butter and beat until fluffy.

Add the eggs, lemon juice, lemon zest and vanilla extract and beat until well combined.

Add the flour mixture and beat until well combined.

Fold in the zucchini and blueberries.

Place the mixture into the prepared loaf pan evenly.

Bake for about 60-70 minutes or until a toothpick inserted in the center comes out clean.

Remove the bread pan from oven and place onto a wire rack to cool for about 10 minutes.

Carefully, invert the bread onto the wire rack to cool completely before slicing.

With a sharp knife, cut the bread loaf into the desired sized slices and serve.

Nutrition:

Calories: 153
Carbohydrates: 5.2g
Protein: 4.5g
Fat: 13.7g
Sugar: 1.7g
Sodium: 87mg
Fiber: 1.9g

19. Multi Seeds Bread

Preparation Time: 1 minutes

Cooking Time: 1 hour

Servings: 16

Ingredients:

1½ C. raw pumpkin seeds, divided

1 C. raw sunflower seeds

½ C. chia seeds

½ C. flax seeds

½ C. psyllium husks

1 tsp. pink Himalayan salt

1/8 tsp. powder stevia

3 C. warm water

3 tbsp. olive oil

Direction:

Preheat the oven to 3500 F. Line a loaf pan with parchment paper.

In a food processor, add 1 C. of pumpkin seeds and pulse until finely ground.

In a large bowl, add the ground pumpkin seed, remaining whole pumpkin seeds, sunflower seeds, chia seeds, flax seeds, psyllium husks, salt and stevia and mix well.

Add the warm water and oil and mix until well combined.

Place the mixture into the prepared bread loaf pan evenly and with your hands, press to smooth the top surface.

Bake for about 45 minutes.

Carefully with the help of the parchment paper, remove the bread loaf from loaf pan.

Arrange the loaf onto a baking sheet, top side down.

Bake for about 15 minutes or until a toothpick inserted in the center comes out clean.

Remove the baking sheet from oven and place onto a wire rack to cool for about 15 minutes.

Carefully, invert the bread onto the wire rack to cool completely before slicing.

With a sharp knife, cut the bread loaf into the desired sized slices and serve.

Nutrition:

Calories: 151
Carbohydrates: 7.9g
Protein: 5.2g
Fat: 12.4g
Sugar: 0.3g
Sodium: 153mg
Fiber: 5.2g

20. Sandwich Bread

Preparation Time: 15 minutes

Cooking Time: 45 minutes

Servings: 16

Ingredients:

2 C. almond flour

1 tsp. organic baking powder

½ tsp. xanthan gum

½ tsp. salt

7 large organic eggs

½ C. butter, melted

2 tbsp. coconut oil

Direction:

Preheat the oven to 3550 F. Line an 8-inch loaf pan with parchment paper.

In a bowl, mix together the almond flour, baking powder, xanthan gum and salt.

In another large bowl, add the eggs and with an electric mixer, beat on high for about 1-2 minutes.

Add the melted butter and coconut oil and beat until smooth.

Add the flour mixture and beat until well combined.

Place the mixture into the prepared loaf pan evenly.

Bake for about 45 minutes or until a toothpick inserted in the center comes out clean.

Remove the bread pan from oven and place onto a wire rack to cool for about 10 minutes.

Carefully, invert the bread onto the wire rack to cool completely before slicing.

With a sharp knife, cut the bread loaf into the desired sized slices and serve.

Nutrition:

Calories: 178
Carbohydrates: 4.4g
Protein: 5.8g
Fat: 16.6g
Sugar: 0.7g
Sodium: 148mg
Fiber: 1.6g

21. Magic Cheese Bread

Preparation Time: 15 minutes

Cooking Time: 17 minutes

Servings: 6

Ingredients:

½ C. almond flour

1 tbsp. Erythritol

1 tbsp. organic baking powder

2 tsp. active dry yeast

2½ C. mozzarella cheese, shredded

2 tbsp. cream cheese, softened

2 large organic eggs, beaten

Directions:

Preheat oven to 4000 F. Line a loaf pan with parchment paper.

In a bowl, mx together the almond flour, Erythritol, yeast and baking powder.

In a microwave-safe bowl, add the mozzarella cheese and cream cheese and microwave for about 1-2 minutes or until melted completely, stirring after every 30 seconds.

Add the flour mixture and mix until well combined.

Add the eggs and mix until a dough ball forms

Place the mixture into the prepared loaf pan evenly.

Bake for about 12-15 minutes or until a toothpick inserted in the center comes out clean.

Remove the bread pan from oven and place onto a wire rack to cool for about 10 minutes.

Carefully, invert the bread onto the wire rack to cool completely before slicing.

With a sharp knife, cut the bread loaf into the desired sized slices and serve.

Nutrition:

Calories: 128
Carbohydrates: 4.3g
Protein: 8.1g
Fat: 9.6g

Sugar: 0.5g
Sodium: 107mg
Fiber: 1.3g

22. 10-Minutes Bread

Preparation Time: 10 minutes

Cooking Time: 10 minutes

Servings: 1

Ingredients:

3 tbsp. almond flour

1 tbsp. butter, melted

½ tsp. organic baking powder

1 large organic egg

Pinch of salt

Direction:

Preheat oven to 3750 F. Lightly, grease an oven safe container.

In a bowl, add all ingredients and mix until well combined.

Place the mixture into the prepared container evenly.

Bake for about 10 minutes or until a toothpick inserted in the center comes out clean.

Remove the bread pan from oven and place onto a wire rack to cool for about 10 minutes.

Carefully, invert the bread onto the wire rack to cool completely before serving.

Nutrition"

Calories: 296
Carbohydrates: 9g
Protein: 10.9g
Fat: 6.1g
Sugar: 1.1g
Sodium: 309mg
Fiber: 2.3g

23. Subtle Rosemary Bread

Preparation Time: 15 minutes

Cooking Time: 50 minutes

Servings: 10

Ingredients:

½ C. coconut flour

1 tsp. organic baking powder

2 tsp. dried rosemary

½ tsp. onion powder

½ tsp. garlic powder

¼ tsp. salt

6 large organic eggs

½ C. butter, melted

Direction:

Preheat oven to 3500 F. Grease an 8x4 loaf pan

In a bowl, mix together the coconut flour, baking powder, rosemary, spices and salt.

In another bowl, add the eggs and with a hand mixer, beat until bubbly.

Slowly, add the butter and beat until smooth.

Slowly, add the flour mixture and beat until well combined.

Place the mixture into the prepared bread loaf pan evenly.

Bake for about 40-50 minutes or until a toothpick inserted in the center comes out clean.

Remove the loaf pan from oven and place onto a wire rack to cool for about 10 minutes.

Carefully, invert the bread onto the wire rack.

With a sharp knife, cut the bread loaf into the desired sized slices and serve warm.

Nutrition:

Calories: 130
Carbohydrates: 1.2g
Protein: 4g
Fat: 12.3g
Sugar: 0.4g
Sodium: 168mg
Fiber: 0.4g

24. Brunch Time Bread

Preparation Time: 15 minutes

Cooking Time: 1 hour

Servings: 10

Ingredients:

7 oz. bacon, chopped

1½ C. almond flour

1 tbsp. organic baking powder

2 organic eggs

1/3 C. sour cream

4 tbsp. butter, melted and cooled

1 C. cheddar cheese, shredded

Direction:

Preheat the oven to 3000 F. Line a loaf pan with greased parchment paper.

Heat a nonstick frying pan over medium heat and cook the bacon for about 8-10 minutes or until crispy.

With a slotted spoon, transfer the bacon onto a plate to drain.

In a bowl, mix together the almond flour and baking powder.

In another bowl, add the eggs and sour cream and beat until smooth.

Add the flour mixture and mix until well combined.

Add the melted butter and mix well.

Gently, fold in the cooked bacon and cheese.

Place the mixture into the prepared bread loaf pan evenly.

Bake for about 45-50 minutes or until a toothpick inserted in the center comes out clean.

Remove the loaf pan from oven and place onto a wire rack to cool for about 10 minutes.

Carefully, invert the bread onto the wire rack.

With a sharp knife, cut the bread loaf into the desired sized slices and serve warm.

Nutrition:

Calories: 321
Carbohydrates: 5.1g
Protein: 15.2g
Fat: 27.6g
Sugar: 0.7g
Sodium: 583mg
Fiber: 1.8g

25. Amazing Cheddar Bread

Preparation Time: 15 minutes

Cooking Time: 45 minutes

Servings: 10

Ingredients:

2 C. almond flour

1 tsp. baking powder

½ tsp. xanthan gum

½ tsp. salt

6 organic eggs

½ C. butter, softened

1½ C. cheddarcheese, shredded and divided

2 tbsp. garlic powder

1 tbsp. parsley flakes

½ tbsp. dried oregano

Direction:

Preheat oven to 3550 F. Line a loaf pan with parchment paper.

In a bowl, mix together the flour, baking powder, xanthan gum and salt.

In another bowl, add the eggs and beat until frothy

Add the butter and mix well.

Slowly, add the flour mixture and mix well.

Add 1 C. of cheese, garlic powder, parsley and oregano and mix well.

Place the mixture into the prepared bread loaf pan evenly and top with the remaining cheese.

Bake for about 45 minutes or until a toothpick inserted in the center comes out clean.

Remove the loaf pan from oven and place onto a wire rack to cool for about 10 minutes.

Carefully, invert the bread onto the wire rack.

With a sharp knife, cut the bread loaf into the desired sized slices and serve warm.

Nutrition:

Calories: 323
Carbohydrates: 7g
Protein: 12.8g
Fat: 28.7g
Sugar: 1.5g
Sodium: 328mg
Fiber: 2.9g

Keto Vegetables Recipes

26. Grain-Free Creamy Noodles

Preparation Time: 15 minutes

Cooking Time: 10 minutes

Servings: 4

Ingredients:

1 ¼ C. heavy whipping cream

¼ C. mayonnaise

Salt and freshly ground black pepper, to taste

30 oz. zucchini, spiralized with blade C

4 organic egg yolks

3 oz. Parmesan cheese, grated

2 tbsp. fresh parsley, chopped

2 tbsp. butter, melted

Direction:

In a pan, add the heavy cream and bring to a boil.

Reduce the heat to low and cook until reduced.

Add the mayonnaise, salt and black pepper and cook until mixture is warm enough.

Add the zucchini noodles and gently, stir to combine.

Immediately, remove from the heat.

Place the zucchini noodles mixture onto 4 serving plates evenly and immediately, top with the egg yolks, followed by the parmesan and parsley.

Drizzle with hot melted butter and serve.

Nutrition:

Calories: 427
Carbohydrates: 9g
Protein: 13g
Fat: 39.1g
Sugar: 3.8g
Sodium: 412mg
Fiber: 2.4g

27. Meat-Free Zoodles Stroganoff

Preparation Time: 20 minutes

Cooking Time: 12 minutes

Servings: 5

Ingredients:

For Mushroom Sauce:

1½ tbsp. butter

1 large garlic clove, minced

1¼ C. fresh button mushrooms, sliced

¼ C. homemade vegetable broth

¼ C. cream

Salt and freshly ground black pepper, to taste

For Zucchini Noodles:

3 large zucchinis, spiralized with blade C

¼ C. fresh parsley leaves, chopped

Direction:

For mushroom sauce: In a large skillet, melt the butter over medium heat and sauté the garlic for about 1 minute.

Stir in the mushrooms and cook for about 6-8 minutes.

Stir in the broth and cook for about 2 minutes, stirring continuously.

Stir in the cream, salt and black pepper and cook for about 1 minute.

Meanwhile, for the zucchini noodles: in a large pan of the boiling water, add the zucchini noodles and cook for about 2-3 minutes.

With a slotted spoon, transfer the zucchini noodles into a colander and immediately rinse under cold running water.

Drain the zucchini noodles well and transfer onto a large paper towel-lined plate to drain.

Divide the zucchini noodles onto serving plates evenly.

Remove the mushroom sauce from the heat and place over zucchini noodles evenly.

Serve immediately with the garnishing of parsley.

Nutrition:

Calories: 77
Carbohydrates: 7.9g
Protein: 3.4g
Fat: 4.6g
Sugar: 4g
Sodium: 120mg
Fiber: 2.4g

28. Eye-Catching Veggies

Preparation Time: 51 minutes

Cooking Time: 20 minutes

Servings: 4

Ingredients:

¼ C. butter

6 scallions, sliced

1 lb. fresh white mushrooms, sliced

1 C. tomatoes, crushed

Salt and freshly ground black pepper, to taste

2 tbsp. feta cheese, crumbled

Direction:

In a large pan, melt the butter over medium-low heat and sauté the scallion for about 2 minutes.

Add the mushrooms and sauté for about 5-7 minutes.

Stir in the tomatoes and cook for about 8-10 minutes, stirring occasionally.

Stir in the salt and black pepper and remove from the heat.

Serve with the topping of feta.

Nutrition:

Calories: 160
Carbohydrates: 7.4g
Protein: 5.5g
Fat: 13.5g
Sugar: 3.9g
Sodium: 211mg
Fiber: 2.3g

29. Favorite Punjabi Curry

Preparation Time: 15 minutes

Cooking Time: 35 minutes

Servings: 3

Ingredients:

1 tbsp. olive oil

½ of small yellow onion, chopped finely

2 small garlic cloves, minced

½ tsp. fresh ginger root, minced

1 small Serrano pepper, seeded and minced

1 tsp. curry powder

¼ tsp. cayenne pepper

1 medium plum tomato, chopped finely

1 large eggplant, cubed

Salt, to taste

¾ C. unsweetened coconut milk

1 tbsp. fresh parsley, chopped

Direction:

In a large skillet, heat the oil over medium heat and sauté the onion for about 6 minutes.

Add the garlic, ginger, Serrano pepper and spices and sauté for about 1 minute.

Add the tomato and cook for about 3 minutes, crushing with the back of a spoon.

Add the eggplant and salt and cook for about 1 minute, stirring occasionally.

Stir in the coconut milk and bring to a gentle boil.

Reduce the heat to medium-low and simmer, covered for about 20 minutes or until done completely.

Serve with the garnishing of the parsley.

Nutrition:

Calories: 105
Carbohydrates: 12g
Protein: 2.1g
Fat: 6.1g
Sugar: 5.2g
Sodium: 57mg
Fiber: 6.6g

30. Traditional Indian Curry

Preparation Time: 15 minutes

Cooking Time: 35 minutes

Servings: 4

Ingredients:

3 tbsp. butter

7 oz. cottage cheese, cut into 2-inch cubes

½ head cauliflower, cut into small florets

½ C. water

1 C. fresh cream

½ C. plain Greek yogurt

1-2 tbsp. curry paste

2 tbsp. fresh cilantro

Direction:

In a large skillet, melt half of the butter over medium heat and stir fry the cottage cheese cubes for about 4-5 minutes or until golden from all sides.

With a slotted spoon, transfer the cheese cubes onto a plate and set aside.

In the same pan, melt the remaining butter and cook the cauliflower for about 2-3 minutes, stirring frequently.

Stir in the water and cook, covered for about 4-5 minutes until all the liquid is absorbed.

Meanwhile, place the cream, yogurt and curry paste in a bowl and beat until smooth.

Stir the yogurt mixture into the frying pan and simmer for about 15-20 minutes, stirring occasionally.

Stir in the fried cheese cubes and cook for about 2 minutes or until heated through.

Garnish with fresh cilantro and serve hot.

Nutrition:

Calories: 215
Carbohydrates: 8.1g
Protein: 10g
Fat: 15.5g
Sugar: 4.3g
Sodium: 315mg
Fiber: 0.9g

31. Vinegar Braised Cabbage

Cooking Time: 30 minutes

Preparation Time: 15 minutes

Servings: 6

Ingredients:

2 tbsp. butter

½ head green cabbage, cut into ¼-inch slices

½ of yellow onion, sliced thinly

1 C. water

1 tbsp. Swerve

1 tbsp. organic apple cider vinegar

2 tsp. caraway seeds

Salt, to taste

Direction:

In a large nonstick skillet, melt the butter over medium heat and sauté the cabbage, garlic and onion for about 5 minutes.

Add the remaining ingredients and stir to combine.

Immediately, reduce the heat to low and simmer for about 20-25 minutes.

Serve warm.

Nutrition:

Calories: 56
Carbohydrates: 5g
Protein: 1g
Fat: 4g
Sugar: 2.3g
Sodium: 67mg
Fiber: 2g

32. Green Veggies Curry

Cooking Time: 25 minutes

Preparation Time: 15 minutes

Servings: 2

Ingredients:

3 tbsp. coconut oil, divided

¼ of small yellow onion, chopped

1 tsp. garlic, minced

1 tsp. fresh ginger, minced

1 C. broccoli florets

1 tbsp. red curry paste

2 C. fresh spinach, torn

½ C. coconut cream

2 tsp. low-sodium soy sauce

2 tsp. red boat fish sauce

¼ tsp. red pepper flakes, crushed

1 tsp. fresh parsley, chopped finely

Direction:

In a large skillet, melt 2 tbsp. of the coconut oil over medium-high heat and sauté the onion for about 3-4 minutes.

Add the garlic and ginger and sauté for about 1 minute.

Add the broccoli and stir to combine well.

Immediately, reduce the heat to medium-low and cook or about 1-2 minutes, stirring continuously.

Stir in the curry paste and cook for about 1 minute, stirring continuously.

Stir in the spinach and cook or about 2 minutes, stirring frequently.

Add the coconut cream and remaining coconut oil and stir until smooth.

Stir in the soy sauce, fish sauce and red pepper flakes and simmer for about 5-10 minutes, stirring occasionally or until the desired thickness of the curry.

Remove from the heat and serve hot with the topping of parsley.

Nutrition:

Calories: 324
Carbohydrates: 11g
Protein: 5.5g
Fat: 30.5g
Sugar: 3.7g
Sodium: 1200mg
Fiber: 3.6g

33. Fuss-Free Veggies Bake

Cooking Time: 20 minutes

Preparation Time: 15 minutes

Servings: 6

Ingredients:

1 large zucchini, chopped

1 large yellow squash, chopped

1 medium green bell pepper, seeded and cubed

1 medium red bell pepper, seeded and cubed

1 yellow onion, sliced thinly

2 tbsp. olive oil

2 tsp. curry powder

1 tsp. ground cumin

½ tsp. paprika

Salt and freshly ground black pepper, to taste

¼ C. homemade vegetable broth

¼ C. fresh cilantro, chopped

Direction:

Preheat the oven to 375 degrees F. Lightly, grease a large baking dish.

In a large bowl, add all the ingredients except cilantro and mix until well combined.

Transfer the vegetable mixture into the prepared baking dish and spread evenly.

Bake for about 15-20 minutes or until the desired doneness of the vegetables.

Remove from the oven and serve immediately with the garnishing of the cilantro.

Nutrition:

Calories: 83
Carbohydrates: 9g
Protein: 2.3g
Fat: 5.2g
Sugar: 4.7g
Sodium: 73mg
Fiber: 2.5g

34.4 Veggies Combo

Cooking Time: 12 minutes

Preparation Time: 20 minutes

Servings: 5

Ingredients:

4 tbsp. butter

½ tsp. fresh ginger, minced

2 large garlic cloves, minced

1½ C. broccoli florets

1 C. carrot, peeled and julienned

1 tbsp. water

8 fresh shiitake mushrooms, sliced

1 C. canned water chestnuts, drained and sliced

1 tsp. arrowroot starch

3 tbsp. homemade vegetable broth

3 tbsp. low-sodium soy sauce

½ tsp. red pepper flakes, crushed

Freshly ground black pepper, to taste

2 tsp. black sesame seeds, toasted

Direction:

In a large skillet, melt the butter over medium-high heat and sauté the ginger and garlic for about 1 minute.

Add the broccoli, carrot and water and cook for about 3-4 minutes.

Add the remaining vegetables and cook for about 2 minutes.

Meanwhile, in a bowl, add the arrowroot starch, broth and soy sauce and mix until well combined.

In the skillet, slowly add the broth mixture, stirring continuously until well combined.

Stir in the red pepper flakes and cook for about 3-4 minutes or until the desired doneness of the vegetables, stirring continuously.

Stir in the black pepper and remove from the heat.

Serve hot with the topping of the sesame seeds.

Nutrition:

Calories: 118
Carbohydrates: 8.4g
Protein: 2.9g
Fat: 8.4g
Sugar: 2.3g
Sodium: 549mg
Fiber: 1.8g

35. Midweek Veggie Supper

Cooking Time: 15 minutes

Preparation Time: 10 minutes

Servings: 4

Ingredients:

2 tbsp. unsalted butter

1 medium yellow onion, chopped

1 C. cream cheese, softened

2 (10-oz.) packages frozen spinach, thawed and squeezed dry

2-3 tbsp. water

Salt and freshly ground black pepper, to taste

2 tsp. fresh lemon juice

Direction:

In a skillet, melt the butter over medium heat and sauté the onion for about 6-8 minutes.

Add the cream cheese and cook for about 2 minutes or until melted completely.

Stir in the spinach and water and cook for about 4-5 minutes.

Stir in the salt, black pepper and lemon juice and remove from heat.

Serve immediately.

Nutrition:

Calories: 298
Carbohydrates: 9g
Protein: 8.8g

Fat: 26.6g
Sugar: 1.9g
Sodium: 365mg
Fiber: 3.7g

36. Buttery Veggies

Cooking Time: 10 minutes

Preparation Time: 15 minutes

Servings: 5

Ingredients:

3 tbsp. butter

4 small garlic cloves, minced

1 large white onion, sliced

3 large red bell peppers, seeded and sliced

2 C. small broccoli florets

¼ C. homemade vegetable broth

Salt and freshly ground white pepper, to taste

Direction:

In a large skillet, heat the oil over medium heat and sauté the garlic for about 1 minute.

Add the vegetables and stir fry for about 5 minutes.

Stir in the broth and stir fry for about 4 minutes or until the desired doneness of the vegetables.

Stir in the salt and white pepper and remove from the heat.

Serve hot.

Nutrition:

Calories: 111
Carbohydrates: 10g
Protein: 2.4g
Fat: 7.3g
Sugar: 5g
Sodium: 133mg
Fiber: 2.5g

37. Best Tasting Kabobs

Cooking Time: 10 minutes

Preparation Time: 20 minutes

Servings: 5

Ingredients:

For Marinade:

2 garlic cloves, minced

2 tsp. fresh basil, minced

2 tsp. fresh oregano, minced

½ tsp. cayenne pepper

Salt and freshly ground black pepper, to taste

2 tbsp. fresh lemon juice

2 tbsp. olive oil

For Veggies:

2 large zucchinis, cut into thick slices

10 large button mushrooms, quartered

1 yellow bell pepper, seeded and cubed

1 red bell pepper, seeded and cubed

Direction:

For marinade: in a large bowl, add all the ingredients and mix until well combined.

Add the vegetables and toss to coat well.

Cover the bowl and refrigerate to marinate for at least 3-4 hours.

Preheat the grill to medium-high heat. Generously, grease the grill grate.

Remove the vegetables from the bowl and thread onto pre-soaked wooden skewers.

Grill for about 8-10 minutes or until done completely, flipping occasionally.

Remove from the grill and place onto a platter for about 5 minutes before serving.

Nutrition:

Calories: 94
Carbohydrates: 9.1g
Protein: 3.6g
Fat: 6.2g
Sugar: 4.4g
Sodium: 50mg
Fiber: 3.1g

Keto Soup & Stew Recipes

38. Winter Comfort stew

Cooking Time: 50 minutes

Preparation Time: 15 minutes

Servings: 6

Ingredients:

2 tbsp. olive oil

1 small yellow onion, chopped

2 garlic cloves, chopped

2 lb. grass-fed beef chuck, cut into 1-inch cubes

1 (14-oz.) can sugar-free crushed tomatoes

2 tsp. ground allspice

1½ tsp. red pepper flakes

½ C. homemade beef broth

6 oz. green olives, pitted

8 oz. fresh baby spinach

2 tbsp. fresh lemon juice

Salt and freshly ground black pepper, to taste

¼ C. fresh cilantro, chopped

Direction:

In a pan, heat the oil in a pan over high heat and sauté the onion and garlic for about 2-3 minutes.

Add the beef and cook for about 3-4 minutes or until browned, stirring frequently.

Add the tomatoes, spices and broth and bring to a boil.

Reduce the heat to low and simmer, covered for about 30-40 minutes or until desired doneness of the beef.

Stir in the olives and spinach and simmer for about 2-3 minutes.

Stir in the lemon juice, salt and black pepper and remove from the heat.

Serve hot with the garnishing of cilantro.

Nutrition:

Calories: 388
Carbohydrates: 8g
Protein: 485g
Fat: 17.7g
Sugar: 2.6g
Sodium: 473mg
Fiber: 3.1g

39. Ideal Cold Weather Stew

Cooking Time: 2 hours 40 minutes

Preparation Time: 20 minutes

Servings: 6

Ingredients:

3 tbsp. olive oil, divided

8 oz. fresh mushrooms, quartered

1¼ lb. grass-fed beef chuck roast, trimmed and cubed into 1-inch size

2 tbsp. tomato paste

½ tsp. dried thyme

1 bay leaf

5 C. homemade beef broth

6 oz. celery root, peeled and cubed

4 oz. yellow onions, chopped roughly

3 oz. carrot, peeled and sliced

2 garlic cloves, sliced

Salt and freshly ground black pepper, to taste

Direction:

In a Dutch oven, heat 1 tbsp. of the oil over medium heat and cook the mushrooms for about 2 minutes, without stirring.

Stir the mushroom and cook for about 2 minutes more.

With a slotted spoon, transfer the mushroom onto a plate.

In the same pan, heat the remaining oil over medium-high heat and sear the beef cubes for about 4-5 minutes.

Stir in the tomato paste, thyme and bay leaf and cook for about 1 minute.

Stir in the broth and bring to a boil.

Reduce the heat to low and simmer, covered for about 1½ hours.

Stir in the mushrooms, celery, onion, carrot and garlic and simmers for about 40-60 minutes.

Stir in the salt and black pepper and remove from the heat.

Serve hot.

Nutrition:

Calories: 447
Carbohydrates: 7.4g
Protein: 30.8g
Fat: 32.3g
Sugar: .8g
Sodium: 764mg
Fiber: 1.9g

40. Weekend Dinner Stew

Cooking Time: 55 minutes

Preparation Time: 15 minutes

Servings: 6

Ingredients:

1½ lb. grass-fed beef stew meat, trimmed and cubed into 1-inch size

Salt and freshly ground black pepper, to taste

1 tbsp. olive oil

1 C. homemade tomato puree

4 C. homemade beef broth

2 C. zucchini, chopped

2 celery ribs, sliced

½ C. carrots, peeled and sliced

2 garlic cloves, minced

½ tbsp. dried thyme

1 tsp. dried parsley

1 tsp. dried rosemary

1 tbsp. paprika

1 tsp. onion powder

1 tsp. garlic powder

Direction:

In a large bowl, add the beef cubes, salt and black pepper and toss to coat well.

In a large pan, heat the oil over medium-high heat and cook the beef cubes for about 4-5 minutes or until browned.

Add the remaining ingredients and stir to combine.

Increase the heat to high and bring to a boil.

Reduce the heat to low and simmer, covered for about 40-50 minutes.

Stir in the salt and black pepper and remove from the heat.

Serve hot.

Nutrition:

Calories: 293
Carbohydrates: 8g
Protein: 9.3g
Fat: 10.7g
Sugar: 4g
Sodium: 223mg
Fiber: 2.3g

41. Mexican Pork Stew

Cooking Time: 2 hours 10 minutes

Preparation Time: 15 minutes

Servings: 1

Ingredients:

3 tbsp. unsalted butter

2½ lb. boneless pork ribs, cut into ¾-inch cubes

1 large yellow onion, chopped

4 garlic cloves, crushed

1½ C. homemade chicken broth

2 (10-oz.) cans sugar-free diced tomatoes

1 C. canned roasted poblano chiles

2 tsp. dried oregano

1 tsp. ground cumin

Salt, to taste

¼ C. fresh cilantro, chopped

2 tbsp. fresh lime juice

Direction:

In a large pan, melt the butter over medium-high heat and cook the pork, onions and garlic for about 5 minutes or until browned.

Add the broth and scrape up the browned bits.

Add the tomatoes, poblano chiles, oregano, cumin, and salt and bring to a boil.

Reduce the heat to medium-low and simmer, covered for about 2 hours.

Stir in the fresh cilantro and lime juice and remove from heat.

Serve hot.

Nutrition:

Calories: 288
Carbohydrates: 8.8g
Protein: 39.6g
Fat: 10.1g
Sugar: 4g
Sodium: 283mg
Fiber: 2.8g

42. Hungarian Pork Stew

Cooking Time: 2 hours 20 minutes

Preparation Time: 15 minutes

Servings: 10

Ingredients:

3 tbsp. olive oil

3½ lb. pork shoulder, cut into 4 portions

1 tbsp. butter

2 medium onions, chopped

16 oz. tomatoes, crushed

5 garlic cloves, crushed

2 Hungarian wax peppers, chopped

3 tbsp. Hungarian Sweet paprika

1 tbsp. smoked paprika

1 tsp. hot paprika

½ tsp. caraway seeds

1 bay leaf

1 C. homemade chicken broth

1 packet unflavored gelatin

2 tbsp. fresh lemon juice

Pinch of xanthan gum

Salt and freshly ground black pepper, to taste

Description:

In a heavy-bottomed pan, heat 1 tbsp. of oil over high heat and sear the pork for about 2-3 minutes or until browned.

Transfer the pork onto a plate and cut into bite-sized pieces.

In the same pan, heat 1 tbsp. of oil and butter over medium-low heat and sauté the onions for about 5-6 minutes.

With a slotted spoon transfer the onion into a bowl.

In the same pan, add the tomatoes and cook for about 3-4 minutes, without stirring.

Meanwhile, in a small frying pan, heat the remaining oil over-low heat and sauté the garlic, wax peppers, all kinds of paprika and caraway seeds for about 20-30 seconds.

Remove from the heat and set aside.

In a small bowl, mix together the gelatin and broth.

In the large pan, add the cooked pork, garlic mixture, gelatin mixture and bay leaf and bring t0 a gentle boil.

Reduce the heat to low and simmer, covered for about 2 hours.

Stir in the xanthan gum and simmer for about 3-5 minutes.

Stir in the lemon juice, salt and black pepper and remove from the heat.

Serve hot.

Nutrition:

Calories: 529
Carbohydrates: 5.8g
Protein: 38.9g
Fat: 38.5g
Sugar: 2.6g
Sodium: 216mg
Fiber: 2.1g

43. Yellow Chicken Soup

Cooking Time: 25 minutes

Preparation Time: 15 minutes

Servings: 5

Ingredients:

2½ tsp. ground turmeric

1½ tsp. ground cumin

1/8 tsp cayenne pepper

2 tbsp. butter, divided

1 small yellow onion, chopped

2 C. cauliflower, chopped

2 C. broccoli, chopped

4 C. homemade chicken broth

1½ C. water

1 tsp. fresh ginger root, grated

1 bay leaf

2 C. Swiss chard, stemmed and chopped finely

½ C. unsweetened coconut milk

3 (4-oz.) grass-fed boneless, skinless chicken thighs, cut into bite-size pieces

2 tbsp. fresh lime juice

Direction:

In a small bowl, mix together the turmeric, cumin and cayenne pepper and set aside.

Ina large pan, melt 1 tbsp. of the butter over medium heat and sauté the onion for about 3-4 minutes.

Add the cauliflower, broccoli and half of the spice mixture and cook for another 3-4 minutes.

Add the broth, water, ginger and bay leaf and bring to a boil.

Reduce the heat to low and simmer for about 8-10 minutes.

Stir in the Swiss chard and coconut milk and cook for about 1-2 minutes.

Meanwhile, in a large skillet, melt the remaining butter over medium heat and sear the chicken pieces for about 5 minutes.

Stir in the remaining spice mix and cook for about 5 minutes, stirring frequently.

Transfer the soup into serving bowls and top with the chicken pieces.

Drizzle with lime juice and serve.

Nutrition:

Calories: 258
Carbohydrates: 8.4g
Protein: 18.4g
Fat: 16.8g
Sugar: 3g
Sodium: 753mg
Fiber: 2.9g

44. Curry Soup

Preparation Time: 25 minutes

Cooking Time: 20 minutes

Servings: 4

Ingredients: ¾ tsp. cumin

¼ c. pumpkin seeds, raw

½ tsp. garlic powder

½ tsp. paprika ½ tsp. sea salt

1 c. coconut milk, unsweetened

1 clove garlic, minced

1 med. onion, diced

2 c. carrots, chopped

2 tbsp. curry powder

3 c. cauliflower, riced

3 tbsp. extra virgin olive oil, divided

4 c. kale, chopped

4 c. vegetable broth

Sea salt & pepper to taste

Direction: Hear a large saute pan over medium heat with 2 tablespoons of olive oil. Once the oil is hot, add the riced cauliflower to the pan along with the curry powder, cumin, salt, paprika, and garlic powder. Stir thoroughly to combine.

While cooking, stir occasionally. Once the cauliflower is warmed through, remove it from the heat.

In a large pot over medium heat, add the remainder of your olive oil. Once it's hot, add the onion and allow it to cook for about four minutes. Add the garlic, then cook for about another two minutes.

To the large pot, add the broth, kale, carrots, and cauliflower. Stir to thoroughly incorporate.

Allow the mixture to come to a boil, drop the heat to low, and allow the soup to simmer for about 15 minutes.

Stir the coconut milk into the mixture along with salt and pepper to taste.

Garnish with pumpkin seeds and serve hot!

Nutrition: Calories: 274

Carbs: 11 grams
Fat 19 grams
Protein 15 grams

45. Delicious Tomato Basil Soup

Preparation Time: 10 minutes

Cook Time: 40 minutes

Servings: 4

Ingredients:

¼ c. olive oil

½ c. heavy cream

1 lb. tomatoes, fresh

4 c. chicken broth, divided

4 cloves garlic, fresh

Sea salt & pepper to taste

Direction:

Preheat oven to 400° Fahrenheit and line a baking sheet with foil.

Remove the cores from your tomatoes and place them on the baking sheet along with the cloves of garlic.

Drizzle tomatoes and garlic with olive oil, salt, and pepper.

Roast at 400° Fahrenheit for 30 minutes.

Pull the tomatoes out of the oven and place into a blender, along with the juices that have dripped onto the pan during roasting.

Add two cups of the chicken broth to the blender.

Blend until smooth, then strain the mixture into a large saucepan or a pot.

While the pan is on the stove, whisk the remaining two cups of broth and the cream into the soup.

Simmer for about ten minutes.

Season to taste, then serve hot!

Nutrition:

Calories: 225
Carbohydrates: 5.5 grams
Fat: 20 grams
Protein: 6.5 grams

46. Chicken Enchilada Soup

Preparation Time: 10 minutes

Cooking Time: 45 minutes

Servings: 4

Ingredients:

½ c. fresh cilantro, chopped

1 ¼ tsp. chili powder

1 c. fresh tomatoes, diced

1 med. yellow onion, diced

1 sm. red bell pepper, diced

1 tbsp. cumin, ground

1 tbsp. extra virgin olive oil

1 tbsp. lime juice, fresh

1 tsp. dried oregano

2 cloves garlic, minced

2 lg. stalks celery, diced

4 c. chicken broth

8 oz. chicken thighs, boneless & skinless, shredded

8 oz. cream cheese, softened

Direction:

1. In a pot over medium heat, warm olive oil.

2. Once hot, add celery, red pepper, onion, and garlic. Cook for about 3 minutes or until shiny.

3. Stir the tomatoes into the pot and let cook for another 2 minutes.

4. Add seasonings to the pot, stir in chicken broth and bring to a boil.

5. Once boiling, drop the heat down to low and allow to simmer for 20 minutes.

6. Once simmered, add the cream cheese and allow the soup to return to a boil.*

7. Drop the heat once again and allow to simmer for another 20 minutes.

8. Stir the shredded chicken into the soup along with the lime juice and the cilantro.

9. Spoon into bowls and serve hot!

Nutrition: Calories: 420
Carbohydrates: 9 grams
Fat: 29.5 grams
Protein: 27 grams

47. Buffalo Chicken Soup

Preparation Time: 20 minutes

Cook Time: 20 minutes

Servings: 4

Ingredients:

4 med. stalks celery, diced

2 med. carrots, diced

4 chicken breasts, boneless & skinless

6 tbsp. butter

1 qt. chicken broth

2 oz. cream cheese

½ c. heavy cream

½ c. buffalo sauce 1 tsp. sea salt

½ tsp. thyme, dried

For garnish:

Sour cream

Green onions, thinly sliced

Bleu cheese crumbles

Direction: Set a large pot to warm over medium heat with the olive oil in it. Cook celery and carrot until shiny and tender. Add chicken breasts to the pot and cover. Allow to cook about five to six minutes per side. Once the chicken has cooked and formed some caramelization on each side, remove it from the pot.

Shred the chicken breasts and set aside. Pour the chicken broth into the pot with the carrots and celery, then stir in the cream, butter, and cream cheese.* Bring the pot to a boil, then add chicken back to the pot. Stir buffalo sauce into the mix and combine completely. Feel free to increase or decrease as desired.

Add seasonings, stir, and drop the heat to low. Allow the soup to simmer for 15 to 20 minutes, or until all the flavors have fully combined. Serve hot with a garnish of sour cream, bleu cheese crumbles, and sliced green onion!

Nutrition:

Calories: 563
Carbohydrates: 4 grams
Fat: 32.5 grams
Protein: 57 grams

48. Slow Cooker Taco Soup

Preparation Time: 10 minutes

Cooking Time: 2 hours

Servings: 8

Ingredients: ¼ c. sour cream

½ c. cheddar cheese, shredded

2 c. diced tomatoes

2 lbs. ground beef

3 tbsp. taco seasoning*

4 c. chicken broth

8 oz. cream cheese, cubed**

Direction:

Heat a medium saucepan over medium heat and brown the beef.

Drain the fat from the beef and then place it into the slow cooker.

Add the cream cheese cubes, taco seasoning, and diced tomatoes into the slow cooker.

Add the chicken broth, cover and leave to cook on high for two hours.

Once the timer is up, stir all the ingredients and spoon the soup into bowls.

Serve hot with sour cream and shredded cheese on top!

*Check the label! Make sure that the taco seasoning you buy doesn't contain hidden sugars or starches.

**Cream cheese is easier to cut when it's very cold and if you carefully spread a little bit of olive oil on the blade of the knife!

Nutrition:

Calories: 505
Carbohydrates: 8.5 grams
Fat: 31.5 grams
Protein: 43.5 grams

49. Wedding Soup

Preparation Time: 5 minutes

Cooking Time: 10 minutes

Servings: 4

Ingredients:

½ c. almond flour

½ c. parmesan cheese, grated

½ sm. yellow onion, diced

1 lb. ground beef

1 lg. egg, beaten

1 tsp. Italian seasoning

1 tsp. oregano, fresh & chopped

1 tsp. thyme, fresh & chopped

2 c. baby leaf spinach, fresh

2 c. cauliflower, riced

2 med. stalks celery, diced

2 tbsp. extra virgin olive oil

3 cloves garlic, minced

6 c. chicken broth

Sea salt & pepper to taste

Direction:

In a large mixing bowl, combine almond flour, parmesan cheese, ground beef, egg, salt, pepper, and Italian seasoning. Mix thoroughly by band

Shape the meat mixture into one-inch meatballs, cover, and refrigerate until ready to cook.

In a large saucepan over medium heat, warm the olive oil.

Once the oil is hot, stir the celery and onion into the pan and season to taste with salt and pepper.

Stirring often, bring the onion and celery to a lightly cooked state, about six or seven minutes.

Add the garlic to the pan, stir to combine, and allow to cook for one more minute.

Stir chicken broth, fresh oregano, and the fresh thyme into the pan and stir to combine.

Bring the mixture to a boil.

Drop the heat to low and allow to simmer for about ten minutes before adding cauliflower and meatballs to it.

Allow to cook for about five minutes or until the meatballs are cooked all the way through.

Add the spinach to the soup and stir in for about one to two minutes, or until it's sufficiently wilted.

Add seasoning as is needed.

Serve hot!

Nutrition:

Calories: 420
Carbohydrates: 4 grams
Fat: 26 grams
Protein: 6.5 grams

50. Slow Cooker Taco Soup

Preparation Time: 10 minutes

Cooking Time: 2 hours

Servings: 8

Ingredients:

¼ c. sour cream

½ c. cheddar cheese, shredded

2 c. diced tomatoes

2 lbs. ground beef

3 tbsp. taco seasoning*

4 c. chicken broth

8 oz. cream cheese, cubed**

Direction:

Heat a medium saucepan over medium heat and brown the beef.

Drain the fat from the beef and then place it into the slow cooker.

Add the cream cheese cubes, taco seasoning, and diced tomatoes into the slow cooker.

Add the chicken broth, cover and leave to cook on high for two hours.

Once the timer is up, stir all the ingredients and spoon the soup into bowls.

Serve hot with sour cream and shredded cheese on top!

*Check the label! Make sure that the taco seasoning you buy doesn't contain hidden sugars or starches.

**Cream cheese is easier to cut when it's very cold and if you carefully spread a little bit of olive oil on the blade of the knife! d

Nutrition: Calories: 505
Carbohydrates: 8.5 grams
Fat: 31.5 grams
Protein: 43.5 grams

Keto Snack Recipes

51. Keto Fat Bombs

Preparation Time: 5 minutes

Cooking Time: 30 minutes

Servings: 8

Ingredients:

¼ tsp. erythritol or equal measure of preferred sweetener

½ c. sugar-free chocolate chips.

½ c. sugar-free peanut butter

5 oz. coconut oil

8 oz. cream cheese, softened

Direction:

Line a baking sheet with parchment paper and set aside.

In a medium bowl, combine cream cheese, peanut butter, sweetener, and four ounces of the coconut oil. Using a hand mixer, create a smooth mixture.

Place the bowl into the freezer for 10 to 15 minutes to allow the "dough" to firm up a little.

Once the dough has become firmer, use a small spoon to separate small bits of dough and roll them into balls. Place the bombs on the baking sheet and place into the refrigerator to stiffen. In a small bowl, combine chocolate chips and remaining coconut oil and het up in the microwave for 30-second intervals. Stir in between each and, once the mixture is fully smooth, drizzle it over the bombs. Place the bombs back in the refrigerator to allow the drizzle to harden.

Store in the refrigerator for future snacking!

Nutrition:

Calories: 290
Carbohydrates: 5 grams
Fat: 28 grams
Protein: 5 grams

52. Asparagus Fries with Dipping Sauce

Preparation Time: 15 minutes

Cooking Time: 15 minutes

Servings: 4

Ingredients: ¼ c. almond flour

½ c. parmesan cheese, shredded

½ tsp. garlic powder

½ tsp. paprika 1 c. mayonnaise

1 tbsp. tomato paste

1 tsp. chipotle powder (increase or decrease according to heat tolerance)

2 lg. eggs, beaten

2 tbsp. parsley, fresh & chopped

24 med. spears asparagus, trimmed

Direction: In a small bowl, combine tomato paste, mayonnaise, and chipotle powder. Whisk until completely smooth and chill until ready to use.

Preheat the oven to 425° Fahrenheit and line a baking sheet with parchment paper.

In a food processor, combine parsley, parmesan cheese, and garlic powder. Pulse until thoroughly combined. Add the almond flour and paprika to the processor and pulse until fully combined.

Empty the food processor into a shallow dish.

Beat eggs and pour into shallow dish. Coat the asparagus spears in egg, then dredge in the almond flour mixture.

Place each spear on the baking sheet in one even layer. Top the spears with the remaining parmesan cheese.

Bake spears for 10 to 12 minutes or until just tender with a crisp, golden exterior. Let stand for two to five minutes, then serve with the chipotle aioli prepared in step one.

Nutrition:

Calories: 505
Carbohydrates: 4 grams
Fat: 49 grams
Protein: 7 grams

53. Bacon-Wrapped Jalapeño Poppers

Preparation Time: 10 minutes

Cooking Time: 30 minutes

Servings: 4

Ingredients:

2 oz. cream cheese, softened

6 oz. ground beef

8 jalapeños, fresh, halved, & seeded

8 slices bacon, halved

Sea salt & pepper to taste

Direction:

Preheat the oven to 400° Fahrenheit and place a wire rack inside baking sheet.

In a large skillet over medium heat, brown the beef, breaking it up into small pieces as it cooks. Season to taste with salt and pepper.

Spoon cream cheese into the halves of each pepper, leaving a little room.

Spoon ground beef into the halves of each pepper.

Wrap the halves of each pepper with a half strip of bacon each.

Place poppers on the rack and bake for 30 minutes. The bacon should crisp on the outside.

Serve warm!

Nutrition:

Calories: 140
Carbohydrates: .5 grams
Fat: 10 grams
Protein: 1 gram

54. Pumpkin Roll Fat Bombs

Preparation Time: 20 minutes

Cooking Time: 0 Minutes

Servings: 12

Ingredients:

For the Bombs:

¼ c. pumpkin puree

½ c. almond butter

½ c. erythritol or comparable measure of preferred sweetener

½ tbsp. pumpkin pie spice

1 tsp. vanilla extract

8 oz. cream cheese, softened

For the Topping:

½ tsp. vanilla extract

1 pinch cinnamon, ground

1 tbsp. erythritol or comparable measure of preferred sweetener

2 oz. cream cheese, softened

2 tbsp. heavy cream

Direction:

Line a baking sheet with parchment paper and set aside.

In a mixing bowl, place softened cream cheese for the bombs and beat with a hand mixer until a fluffy texture is achieved.

Add almond butter, sweetener, and puree and mix to combine completely. Add pumpkin pie spice and vanilla, then mix once more.

Chill the mixture in the refrigerator for 30 minutes (or the freezer for 15) to firm up the "dough."

Using a spoon, take small pieces of the dough out of the bowl one at a time and roll them into balls. As you're done rolling them, place each one onto the baking sheet.

Place the baking sheet into the freezer for about 45 minutes to firm them up.

In a mixing bowl, combine all ingredients for the topping and beat with hand mixer until well combined.

Top the bombs with the topping, dust with cinnamon and serve!

These can be stored in the refrigerator for future snacking!

Nutrition:

Calories: 100
Carbohydrates: 1 gram, Fat: 10 grams
Protein: 2 grams

55. Smoked Salmon Dip

Preparation Time: 10 minutes

Cooking Time: 0 minutes

Servings: 12

Ingredients:

½ c. sour cream

½ tsp. black pepper

½ tsp. sea salt

1 ½ tbsp. lemon juice, fresh

1 tbsp. dill, fresh & chopped

4 oz. salmon, smoked & minced

8 oz. cream cheese, softened

Direction:

In a small mixing bowl, beat the cream cheese with a hand mixer until soft and creamy.

Add fill, lemon juice, salt, pepper, and sour cream, then beat once again to thin and smooth the mixture.

Using a spoon, mix the salmon into the dip until fully combined.

Chill until ready to serve.

Serve with carrot and celery sticks!

Nutrition:

Calories: 100
Carbohydrates: 1 gram, Fat: 9 grams
Protein: 3.5 grams

56. Chewy Granola Bars

Preparation Time: 10 minutes

Cooking Time: 25 minutes

Servings: 16

Ingredients:

½ c. butter

½ c. cranberries, dried, unsweetened, & chopped

½ c. erythritol or comparable measure of preferred sweetener

½ c. flaked coconut, unsweetened

½ c. pecans, raw & unsalted

½ c. sunflower seeds, unsalted

½ tsp. vanilla extract

1 ½ c. sliced almonds

1 pinch sea salt

Direction:

Preheat the oven to 300° Fahrenheit and place parchment paper inside baking sheet.

In a food processor, combine almonds, pecans, sunflower seeds, and coconut.

Pulse until the mixture is crumbly like a fine granola.

Place this mixture into a mixing bowl along with cranberries and a pinch of salt, stirring to full incorporate.

In a saucepan over medium heat, warm the butter, then stir in vanilla and sweetener until fully smooth.

Pour the butter mixture over the granola and mix completely to coat.

Press the granola into the baking sheet and form a tight shape with it, about half an inch thick. The tighter it's packed, the better.

Bake for about 25 minutes, then let stand until it's completely cooled.

Cut the baked mix into 16 evenly-sized bars. Store in a dry container and keep for a snack here and there!

Nutrition:

Calories: 180
Carbohydrates: 2 grams
Fat: 17 grams
Protein: 4 grams

57. Almond Butter Fudge Bars

Preparation Time: 25 minutes

Cooking Time: 10 minutes

Servings: 8

Ingredients:

¼ c. heavy cream

½ c. almond butter

½ c. butter, unsalted, melted, & divided

½ tsp. cinnamon, ground

½ tsp. vanilla extract

1 c. almond flour

1 oz. sugar-free chocolate chips

1/8 tsp. xanthan gum

6 tbsp. powdered erythritol or comparable measure of preferred sweetener, divided

Direction:

Preheat the oven to 400° Fahrenheit and place parchment paper inside a medium baking dish.

In a medium mixing bowl, combine one quarter cup melted butter, almond flour, two tablespoons of sweetener, and cinnamon. Mix until all the ingredients are fully combined.

Spread this mixture into the bottom of the dish and press down into one even layer across the bottom.

Bake for 10 minutes and a golden brown color should form on top of it.

Remove from the oven and set aside.

In a medium mixing bowl, combine the heavy cream, remaining melted butter, almond butter, and sweetener. Stir to completely combine.

Pour vanilla extract and xanthan gum into the mixture and stir thoroughly.

Spread the mixture over top of the crust and press it into an even layer.

Sprinkle the chocolate chips onto the top and freeze overnight.

Slice into eight bars and serve, or keep stored for an occasional treat!

Nutrition:

Calories: 235
Carbohydrates: 2 grams
Fat: 24 grams
Protein: 4.5 grams

58. Creamed Spinach Pockets with Apple Slaw

Preparation Time: 35 minutes

Cooking Time: 15 minutes

Servings: 3

Ingredients:

For the Crust:

½ c. almond flour

½ tsp. sea salt 2 lg. eggs, beaten

2/5 c. mozzarella cheese, shredded

6 tbsp. coconut flour

For the Filling:

1 tsp. extra virgin olive oil

¼ c. parmesan cheese, grated

1 pinch sea salt

4 oz. cream cheese, softened

6 oz. spinach, frozen & drained

For the Topping:

¼ c. mayonnaise

¼ tsp. sea salt

¾ c. coleslaw salad mix

1 gala apple, grated

Direction:

Preheat the oven to 350° Fahrenheit and line a baking sheet with parchment paper.

In a medium mixing bowl, combine the coleslaw mix, grated apple, mayonnaise and salt. Stir until everything is completely coated, then cover and refrigerate until ready to serve.

In a large pan over medium heat, warm the olive oil for the filling, then wilt the spinach for three to four minutes. Stir the cream cheese and parmesan into the pan and stir continuously until thoroughly combined. Kill the heat and set the pan aside.

In a small bowl, place mozzarella and microwave at 30-second intervals, stirring in between until the cheese is soft and malleable.

Add the flours to the cheese and stir completely. Add the beaten eggs and salt and mix once more.

Once the mixture is completely mixed, sandwich the dough

between two sheets of parchment paper or wax paper and roll out the dough with a rolling pin. Try to ensure the dough is rolled out to an even thickness the whole way through. Slice the dough into 15 rectangles (or make larger pockets if that suits you and your guests). Spoon the mixture onto the rectangles of dough about ½ a teaspoon at a time (more if your pockets are larger) and fold the dough over to cover the filling. Crimp the sides of the pockets with your fingers so the filling doesn't escape and carefully slice little vents into the tops of each.

Place each completed roll onto the baking sheet and bake for 16 to 18 minutes, or until crisp and golden brown.

Let cool for about five minutes before plating, then spoon slaw over top of the rolls and serve!

Nutrition:

Calories: 670
Carbohydrates: 16 grams
Fat: 67 grams
Protein: 32 grams

59. No-Churn Ice Cream

Preparatio Time: 10 minutes

Cooking Time: 0 minutes

Total Time: 3 hr 10 mins.

Servings: 3

Ingredients:

Pinch salt

1 cup heavy whipping cream

¼ tsp xanthan gum

2 tbsp zero calorie sweetener powder

1 tsp vanilla extract

1 tbsp vodka

Direction:

You'll need an immersion blender and a jar that is pint sized with a wide mouth. First, add the xanthan gum, heavy cream, vanilla extract, sweetener, vodka, and salt to a jar and mix.

Transfer the mixture to the immersion blender and, with the up-down motion, blend until you are left with a thick mixture. This should take up to

2 minutes. Put the mixture back in the jar, cover it, and place it in your freezer for 4 hours. Remember to stir the cream mixture in 40 minutes intervals.

Nutrition:

Calories: 291 Carbs: 3.2g Protein: 1.6g Fat: 29.4g Cholesterol: 109mg Sodium: 92mg

60. Cheesecake Cupcakes

Preparation Time: 10 minutes

Cooking Time: 15 minutes

Total Time: 8 hrs 25 mins.

Servings: 12

Ingredients: 1 tsp vanilla extract ½ cup almond meal

¾ cup granulated no calorie sucralose sweetener ¼ cup melted butter 2 eggs

2 8 oz pack softened cream cheese

Direction:

Preheat your oven to 350 degrees F. Also, prepare 12 muffin cups by lining them with paper liners.Grab a bowl and put your butter and almond meal in it. Using a spoon, take the almond meal mixture and put into the bottom of the muffin cup. Press them down with the flat of the spoon to form a crust.In a separate bowl, add vanilla extract, cream cheese, sucralose sweetener, and eggs. Set an electric mixer to medium and combine the vanilla extract mixture until you get a smooth consistency. Using a spoon, add this mixture to the top of the muffin cups.Pop the muffin cups in the oven and bake until the center of the mixture is slightly set. This should take no more than 17 minutes.Now, you have your cupcakes. Set them aside to cool. When they are safe enough to hold again, put them in your refrigerator. They should stay there 8 hours until the next day, when you can serve them.

Nutrition: Calories: 209 Carbs: 3.5g Protein: 4.9g Fat: 20g Cholesterol: 82mg Sodium: 151mg

61. Brownies

Preparation Time: 10 minutes

Cooking Time: 30 minutes

Total Time: 40 minutes

Servings: 12

Ingredients:

¼ tsp salt

¾ cup cocoa powder

1 tsp vanilla extract

½ tsp baking soda

1 ⅓ cups almond flour

⅔ cup coconut oil, separated

2 eggs

½ cup hot water

1 cup stevia sugar substitute

Direction:

Heat your oven to 350 degrees F before you start. Next, prepare an 8" pan by greasing it with coconut oil.

Get a medium bowl and throw your baking soda and cocoa powder into it. Also, add the hot water and ⅓ cup coconut oil to the bowl. Mix these ingredients properly until you have an even mixture. Now, you can add what is left of your coconut oil, eggs, and stevia. Mix them some more. Lastly, throw some salt, almond flour, and vanilla extract in the mix. Stir the batter well until the ingredients are combined.

Turn this batter onto the pan you had prepared with coconut oil. Next, pop the pan in the oven for about 35 minutes. During this time, the top of the once-batter would have dried. Take the pan out and let it cool.

Use a kitchen knife to cut 12 squares in the large brownie.

Nutrition:

Calories: 222 Carbs: 17.5g Protein: 5g Fat: 20.5g Cholesterol: 31mg Sodium: 114mg

62. Chocolate Peanut Butter Cups

Preparation Time: 15 minutes

Cooking Time: 3 minutes

Total Time: 1 hr 18 mins.

Servings: 12

Ingredients:

1 oz roasted peanuts, chopped and salted

1 cup coconut oil

¼ tsp kosher salt

½ cup natural peanut butter

¼ tsp vanilla extract

2 tbsp heavy cream

1 tsp liquid stevia

1 tbsp cocoa powder

Direction:

You'll need your stove at low heat for this recipe. Place a saucepan on the heat and add coconut oil. After about 5 minutes, add peanut butter, salt, heavy cream, cocoa powder, vanilla extract, and liquid stevia to the pan. Stir till the peanut butter melts.

Get 12 silicone muffin molds and pour the peanut butter mixture in it. Add the salted peanuts on top. Transfer the muffin molds to a baking sheet and place the pan in your freezer. Let it stay in the freezer for an hour, then unmold the cups. Place the chocolate peanut cups in any airtight container.

Nutrition:

Calories: 246 Carbs: 3.3g Protein: 3.4g Fat: 26g Cholesterol: 3mg Sodium: 89mg

63. Peanut Butter Cookies

Preparation Time: 10 minutes

Cooking Time: 15 minutes

Total Time: 25 minutes

Servings: 12

Ingredients:

1 tsp vanilla extract, sugar-free

1 cup peanut butter 1 egg

½ cup natural sweetener, low-calorie

Direction:

Preheat the oven to 350 degrees F for this recipe. Follow that by preparing a baking sheet. Line the sheet using parchment paper.

Into a bowl, add peanut butter, vanilla extract, sweetener, and egg. Mix these ingredients well until you are left with dough.

Using your hands, mold the dough into balls. These balls should be no more than 1 inch in size. Place them on the baking sheet you had prepared and flatten them with a fork. You'll probably love the pattern that forms on the flattened dough. Put the baking sheet in the oven and let the cookies bake for 15 minutes. Afterwards, take the pan out of the oven and just let it sit. After a minute of cooling, it should be safe for you to place on a wire rack to cool even further.

Nutrition:

Calories: 133 Carbs: 12.4g Protein: 5.9g Fat: 11.2g Cholesterol: 16mg Sodium: 105mg

64. Low-Carb Almond Coconut Sandies

Preparation Time: 15 minutes

Cooking Time: 12 minutes

Total Time: 37 minutes

Servings: 18

Ingredients:

⅓ tsp stevia powder

1 cup coconut, unsweetened

1 tsp Himalayan sea salt

1 cup almond meal

1 tbsp vanilla extract

⅓ cup melted coconut oil

2 tbsp water

1 egg white

Direction:

Your oven should be preheated to 325 degrees F before you begin this dish. In addition to that, prepare a baking sheet by lining it with parchment paper.

Get a large bowl and put your Himalayan sea salt, unsweetened coconut, stevia powder, almond meal, vanilla extract, coconut oil, water, and egg white in it. Stir this mixture properly. Set the bowl aside for 10 minutes. This is so that the unsweetened coconut will get considerably softer.

Mold the mixture into little balls. They should be small enough to fit on a tablespoon. Place each ball on the prepared baking sheet. There should be some space between them.

Press down on the balls using a fork. Do this gently, as you don't want the edges to fall off.

Place the baking sheet in your oven and let the Sandies bake for about 15 minutes. After letting the baking sheet cool for a minute, place it on a wire rack to get even cooler.

Nutrition:

Calories: 107 Carbs: 2.7g Protein: 1.9g Fat: 10.5g Cholesterol: 0 mg Sodium: 105mg

65. Creme Brulee

Preparation Time: 10 minutes

Cooking Time: 34 minutes

Total Time: 44 minutes

Servings: 4

Ingredients:

5 tbsp separated natural sweetener, low calorie

4 egg yolks

2 cups heavy whipping cream

1 tsp vanilla extract

Instructions:

Make sure that your oven is preheated to 325 degrees F. Also, get a bowl and put the vanilla extract and egg yolks in it. Use a whisk to mix them properly.

Set your stove to medium heat and put a saucepan on it. Add 1 tbsp of natural sweetener and heavy cream to the pan and mix using a whisk. When you notice the mixture begin to simmer, take the pan down. Get 4 ramekins and separate the mixture equally between them. Place the ramekins in a glass baking dish and add hot water. The water should be an inch to the sides of the ramekins.

Place the glass baking dish at the center of the oven, and leave it there for 30 minutes. By this time, the Creme Brulee should have set. Add 1 tbsp natural sweetener on top of the Creme Brulee.

Here's the really cool part: get a culinary torch and flame the sweetener until it turns a golden color and melts.

Nutrition:

Calorie: 466 Carbs: 16.9g Protein: 5.1g Fat: 48.4g Cholesterol: 368mg Sodium: 53mg

Keto Salad Recipes

66. Chicken avocado salad

Preparation time: 40 minutes

Cooking Time: 0 minutes

Servings: 4

Ingredients:

½ teaspoon pepper

1 pound of boneless chicken thighs

4 tablespoons of extra virgin olive oil

3 tablespoons of chopped celeries

2 tablespoons of cilantro

1 large ripe avocado

1 ½ teaspoon of oregano

1 tablespoon of lemon juice

½ cup almond milk ½ cup diced onion

Direction:

Pour in almond milk in a bowl, add in the oregano, then stir well.

Slice up the boneless chicken thighs, and rub the slices with the almond milk mixture. Let it sit for 13 to 15 minutes.

Preheat an oven to 300°F, and line the baking tray with a foil sheet.

Place the coated chicken slices on the baking tray and bake for 30 to 40 minutes.

Meanwhile, slice the avocado into cubes, then drizzles some olive oil and lemon juice, and set aside.

In a salad bowl, mix in the cilantro, chopped celeries, and onion, and sprinkle some pepper, mix well.

Take out the chicken and garnish with the avocado mix and salad. Serve warm.

Nutrition:

Calories 256g
Total Fat 49g
Total Carbs 8g
 Protein: 19

67. Low carb Caesar salad

Preparation time: 20 minutes

Cooking time: 0 minutes

Servings: 4

Ingredients:

SALAD

1 head of romaine lettuce

6 slices of cooked and diced bacon

½ cup shredded parmesan cheese

DRESSING

5 tablespoons grated parmesan cheese

3 teaspoons Worcestershire sauce

2 teaspoons fresh lemon juice

2 minced anchovy fillets, or anchovy sauce

2/3 cup Keto mayonnaise

¼ cup sour cream

1 minced garlic clove

1 teaspoon mustard powder

Black pepper

Direction:

Slice the lettuce, and mix with cheese and bacon like a normal salad.

For the dressing, put all the ingredients in a single bowl and mix well.

Set down your salad and top with as much dressing as you want. Enjoy!

Nutrition:

Calories: 112
Total Fat: 32g
Total Carbs: 5.0g
 Protein: 14.3g

68. Keto broccoli salad

Preparation time: 20 minutes

Cooking Time: 0 Minutes

Servings: 3

Ingredients:

For the salad:

5 thin slices of bacon

1 ½ head of broccoli, cut into bite-size pieces

½ of a small red onion

¼ cups of shredded Cheddar

¼ of toasted and thinly sliced almonds

1 teaspoon of chopped chives

Kosher salt

Six cups of fat water

For the dressing:

8 small-sliced boneless and skinned chicken breasts

2 tablespoons of apple cider vinegar

1/3 cups of Keto mayonnaise

1 tablespoon of Keto mustard

Black pepper

Kosher salt

Direction:

Cut the broccoli into tiny sizes Add fat water in a pot, add a teaspoon of salt, and let it boil.3

Meanwhile, add iced water in a large pot. When the salted water boils, put in the broccoli florets, and cook for 1-2 minutes.

Take out the broccoli florets and immerse in the ice water for 2 to 3 minutes, then drain.

In another bowl, put in chicken breasts, apple cider vinegar, Keto mayonnaise, Keto mustard, black pepper, a pinch of salt, then toss, and put in a refrigerator. In another bowl, add in the bacon, broccoli, onions, shredded cheddar, almonds, chives, and a pinch of salt for the salad. Toss the refrigerated dressing over the salad before serving.

Nutrition:

Calories: 147

Total Fat: 21g

Total Carbs: 3.5g

Protein: 6.8g

69. Keto chicken-cheese salad

Preparation time: 30 minutes

Cooking Time: 0 Minutes

Servings: 4

Ingredients:

SALAD

½ head of romaine lettuce

6 slices of cooked and diced chicken

2 slices of cooked and diced bacon

½ cup shredded parmesan cheese

DRESSING

5 tablespoons grated parmesan cheese

3 teaspoons Worcestershire sauce

2/3 cup Keto mayonnaise

¼ cup sour cream

1 minced garlic clove

1 teaspoon Keto mustard

Direction:

Slice the lettuce, and toss in the chicken and bacon.

Melt cheese in the microwave, and add in the chicken, lettuce and bacon mixture. Toss well.

For the dressing, put the cheese, sauce, and mayo in a bowl, mix well. Then, add the sour cream, garlic and mustard.

Add the desired amount of dressing in the salad, and enjoy.

Nutrition:

Calories: 103 kcal
Total Fat: 30g
Total Carbs: 4.8g
Protein: 13.9g

70. Keto hamburger salad

Preparation time: 25 minutes

Cooking Time: 0 Minutes

Servings: 3

Ingredients:

1 pound of ground beef

2 cloves of ground garlic

1 onion

3 tablespoons of grass-fed ghee

1 sliced avocado

Arugula

Basil leaf

1 teaspoon of brain octane oil

1 large chopped tomato

1 tablespoon of olive oil

Direction:

Mix in beef, seasoning, and a teaspoon of brain octane oil. Mix well.

Dice onions, and put half of the onions in the meat mixture, mix again.

Shape the meat into patties form.

Heat oil or ghee in a pan on medium heat.

Fry the patties, and let each side brown equally.

Put another pot on the fire, and add olive oil.

Put in your avocado slices, the remaining onions, arugula and basil leaf and sauté the salad for 1 minute.

Place patties and salad in a bowl with chopped tomatoes, and serve.

Nutrition:

Calories: 632 kcal
Total Fat: 43g
Total Carbs: 15g
 Protein: 49g

71. Keto tomato and avocado salad

Preparation time: 15 minutes

Cooking Time: 0 Minutes

Servings: 3

Ingredients:

6 cherry tomatoes

1 small avocado

2 hardboiled eggs

2 cups of mixed green salad

2 pounds of shredded chicken breast

1 ounce of crumbled feta cheese,

½ cup of cooked and crumbled bacon

Direction:

Dice tomatoes, avocadoes and eggs. Toss them in a bowl together.

In another bowl, put the green salad mix, then add the cheese, bacon, and chicken, and mix thoroughly.

Mix in the tomatoes, avocadoes, and egg well.

Nutrition:

Calories: 448 kcal
Total Fat: 40.3g
Total Carbs: 2.8g
Protein: 16.9g

72. Calamari mayo with cauliflower broccoli salad

Preparation time: 30 minutes

Cooking Time: 0 Minutes

Servings: 4-6

Ingredients:

1 ½ pound of fresh squids

1 ½ tablespoon of lemon juice

2 eggs

2 cups of almond flour

2 cups of broccoli florets

2 cups of cauliflower florets

1 cup of extra virgin olive oil

1 diced onion

½ cup diced cheddar cheese

½ cup of mayonnaise

½ teaspoon of pepper

½ cup of sour cream

Direction:

Steam cauliflower and broccoli until they are soft and tender. Set it aside.

Remove squid ink.

Whisk the eggs, and add salt and pepper to taste.

Cut the squid into rings, and put in the egg mixture.

Pour in almond flour, and rub into the squid and egg mix well.

Heat oil in a pan, and fry the squid until it is golden brown.

Take out the squid and set it aside.

In a separate bowl, mix in mayonnaise, lemon juice, and sour cream thoroughly.

To serve, place the fried squid on a plate with the steam broccoli and cauliflower florets, then pour the mayonnaise, lemon juice, and sour cream on it.

Sprinkle dry cheddar cheese on top for garnishing.

Nutrition:

Calories: 452 kcal
Total Fat: 39g
Total Carbs: 5g— Protein: 19.5g

73. Chicken Spinach salad

Preparation time: 15 minutes

Cooking Time: 0 Minutes

Servings: 3

Ingredients:

2 ½ cups of spinach

4 ½ ounces of boiled chicken

2 boiled eggs

½ cup of chopped cucumber

3 slices of bacon

1 small avocado

1 tablespoon olive oil

½ teaspoon of Brain Octane oil

Pinch of Salt

Pepper

Direction:

Dice the boiled eggs.

Slice boiled chicken, bacon, avocado, spinach, and cucumber, and combine them in a bowl. Then add diced boiled eggs.

Drizzle with some oil. Mix well.

Add salt and pepper to taste.

Nutrition:

Calories: 303 kcal
Total Fat: 28.9g
Total Carbs: 4.6g— Protein: 43.3g

Keto Red Meat Recipes

74. Classic Pork Tenderloin

Preparation Time: 15 minutes

Cooking Time: 35 minutes

Servings: 4

Ingredients:

8 bacon slices

2 lb. pork tenderloin

1 tsp. dried oregano, crushed

1 tsp. dried basil, crushed

1 tbsp. garlic powder

1 tsp. seasoned salt

3 tbsp. butter

Directions:

Preheat the oven to 400 degrees F.

Heat a large ovenproof skillet over medium-high heat and cook the bacon for about 6-7 minutes.

Transfer the bacon onto a paper towel lined plate to drain.

Then, wrap the pork tenderloin with bacon slices and secure with toothpicks.

With a sharp knife, slice the tenderloin between each bacon slice to make a medallion.

In a bowl, mix together the dried herbs, garlic powder and seasoned salt.

Now, coat the medallion with herb mixture.

With a paper towel, wipe out the skillet.

In the same skillet, melt the butter over medium-high heat and cook the pork medallion for about 4 minutes per side.

Now, transfer the skillet into the oven.

Roast for about 17-20 minutes.

Remove the wok from oven and let it cool slightly before cutting.

Cut the tenderloin into desired size slices and serve.

Nutrition:

Calories: 471
Carbohydrates: 1g
Protein: 53.5g
Fat: 26.6g
Sugar: 0.1g
Sodium: 1100mg
Fiber: 0.2g

75. Signature Italian Pork Dish

Preparation Time: 15 minutes

Cooking Time: 15 minutes

Servings: 6

Ingredients:

2 lb. pork tenderloins, cut into 1½-inch pieces

¼ C. almond flour

1 tsp. garlic salt

Freshly ground black pepper, to taste

2 tbsp. butter

½ C. homemade chicken broth

1/3 C. balsamic vinegar

1 tbsp. capers

2 tsp. fresh lemon zest, grated finely

Direction:

In a large bowl, add the pork pieces, flour, garlic salt and black pepper and toss to coat well.

Remove pork pieces from bowl and shake off excess flour mixture.

In a large skillet, melt the butter over medium-high heat and cook the pork pieces for about 2-3 minutes per side.

Add broth and vinegar and bring to a gentle boil.

Reduce the heat to medium and simmer for about 3-4 minutes.

With a slotted spoon, transfer the pork pieces onto a plate.

In the same skillet, add the capers and lemon zest and simmer for about 3-5 minutes or until desired thickness of sauce.

Pour sauce over pork pieces and serve.

Nutrition:

Calories: 373
Carbohydrates: 1.8g
Protein: 46.7g
Fat: 18.6g
Sugar: 0.4g
Sodium: 231mg
Fiber: 0.7g

76. Flavor Packed Pork Loin

Preparation Time: 15 minutes

Cooking Time: 1 hour

Servings: 6

Ingredients:

1/3 C. low-sodium soy sauce

¼ C. fresh lemon juice

2 tsp. fresh lemon zest, grated

1 tbsp. fresh thyme, finely chopped

2 tbsp. fresh ginger, grated

2 garlic cloves, chopped finely

2 tbsp. Erythritol

Freshly ground black pepper, to taste

½ tsp. cayenne pepper

2 lb. boneless pork loin

Direction:

For pork marinade: in a large baking dish, add all the ingredients except pork loin and mix until well combined.

Add the pork loin and coat with the marinade generously.

Refrigerate for about 24 hours.

Preheat the oven to 400 degrees F.

Remove the pork loin from marinade and arrange into a baking dish.

Cover the baking dish and bake for about 1 hour.

Remove from the oven and place the pork loin onto a cutting board.

With a piece of foil, cover each loin for at least 10 minutes before slicing.

With a sharp knife, cut the pork loin into desired size slices and serve.

Nutrition:

Calories: 230
Carbohydrates: 3.2g
Protein: 40.8g
Fat: 5.6g
Sugar: 1.2g
Sodium: 871mg
Fiber: 0.6g

77. Spiced Pork Tenderloin

Preparation Time: 15 minutes

Cooking Time: 18 minutes

Servings: 6

Ingredients:

2 tsp. fresh rosemary, minced

2 tsp. fennel seeds

2 tsp. coriander seeds

2 tsp. caraway seeds

1 tsp. cumin seeds

1 bay leaf

Salt and freshly ground black pepper, to taste

2 tbsp. fresh dill, chopped

2 (1-lb.) pork tenderloins, trimmed

Direction:

For spice rub: in a spice grinder, add the seeds and bay leaf and grind until finely powdered.

Add the salt and black pepper and mix.

In a small bowl, reserve 2 tbsp. of spice rub.

In another small bowl, mix together the remaining spice rub, and dill.

Place 1 tenderloin over a piece of plastic wrap.

With a sharp knife, slice through the meat to within ½-inch of the opposite side. Now, open the tenderloin like a book. Cover with another plastic wrap and with a meat pounder, gently pound into ½-inch thickness. Repeat with the remaining tenderloin. Remove the plastic wrap and spread half of the dill mixture over the center of each tenderloin.

Roll each tenderloin like a cylinder.

With a kitchen string, tightly tie each roll at several places.

Rub each roll with the reserved spice rub generously.

With 1 plastic wrap, wrap each roll and refrigerate for at least 4-6 hours.

Preheat the grill to medium-high heat. Grease the grill grate.

Remove the plastic wrap from tenderloins.

Place tenderloins onto the grill and cook for about 14-18 minutes, flipping occasionally.

Remove from the grill and place tenderloins onto a cutting board and with a piece of foil, cover each tenderloin for at least 5-10 minutes before slicing.

With a sharp knife, cut the tenderloins into desired size slices and serve.

Nutrition:

Calories: 313
Carbohydrates: 1.4g
Protein: 45.7g
Fat: 12.6g
Sugar: 0g
Sodium: 127mg
Fiber: 0.7g

78. Sticky Pork Ribs

Preparation Time: 15 minutes

Cooking Time: 2 hours 34 minutes

Servings: 9

Ingredients: ¼ C. Erythritol

1 tbsp. garlic powder

1 tbsp. paprika

½ tsp. red chili powder

4 lb. pork ribs, membrane removed

Salt and freshly ground black pepper, to taste

1½ tsp. liquid smoke

1½ C. sugar-free BBQ sauce

Direction: Preheat the oven to 300 degrees F. Line a large baking sheet with 2 layers of foil, shiny side out. In a bowl, add the Erythritol, garlic powder, paprika and chili powder and mix well.

Season the ribs with salt and black pepper and then, coat with the liquid smoke. Now, rub the ribs with the Erythritol mixture.

Arrange the ribs onto the prepared baking sheet, meaty side down.

Arrange 2 layers of foil on top of ribs and then, roll and crimp edges tightly.

Bake for about 2-2½ hours or until desired doneness.

Remove the baking sheet from oven and place the ribs onto a cutting board.

Now, set the oven to broiler.

With a sharp knife, cut the ribs into serving sized portions and evenly coat with the barbecue sauce.

Arrange the ribs onto a broiler pan, bony side up.

Broil for about 1-2 minutes per side. Remove from the oven and serve hot.

Nutrition:

Calories: 530
Carbohydrates: 2.8g
Protein: 60.4g
Fat: 40.3g
Sugar: 0.4g
Sodium: 306mg
Fiber: 0.5g

79. Valentine's Day Dinner

Preparation Time: 15 minutes

Cooking Time: 35 minutes

Servings: 4

Ingredients:

1 tbsp. olive oil

4 large boneless rib pork chops

1 tsp. salt

1 C. cremini mushrooms, chopped roughly

3 tbsp. yellow onion, chopped finely

2 tbsp. fresh rosemary, chopped

1/3 C. homemade chicken broth

1 tbsp. Dijon mustard

1 tbsp. unsalted butter

2/3 C. heavy cream

2 tbsp. sour cream

Direction:

Heat the oil in a large skillet over medium heat and sear the chops with the salt for about 3-

4 minutes or until browned completely.

With a slotted spoon, transfer the pork chops onto a plate and set aside.

In the same skillet, add the mushrooms, onion and rosemary and sauté for about 3 minutes. Stir in the cooked chops, broth and bring to a boil. Reduce the heat to low and cook, covered for about 20 minutes.

With a slotted spoon, transfer the pork chops onto a plate and set aside. In the skillet, stir in the butter until melted. Add the heavy cream and sour cream and stir until smooth. Stir in the cooked pork chops and cook for about 2-3 minutes or until heated completely.

Serve hot.

Nutrition:

Calories: 400
Carbohydrates: 3.6g
Protein: 46.3g
Fat: 21.6g
Sugar: 0.8g
Sodium: 820mg
Fiber: 1.1g

80. South East Asian Steak Platter

Preparation Time: 15 minutes

Cooking Time: 20 minutes

Servings: 4

Ingredients:

14 oz. grass-fed sirloin steak, trimmed and cut into thin strips

Freshly ground black pepper, to taste

2 tbsp. olive oil, divided

1 small yellow onion, chopped

2 garlic cloves, minced

1 Serrano pepper, seeded and chopped finely

3 C. broccoli florets

3 tbsp. low-sodium soy sauce

2 tbsp. fresh lime juice

Direction:

Season steak with black pepper.

In a large skillet, heat 1 tbsp. of the oil over medium heat and cook the steak for about 6-8 minutes or until browned from all sides.

Transfer the steak onto a plate.

In the same skillet, heat the remaining oil and sauté onion for about 3-4 minutes. Add the garlic and Serrano pepper and sauté for about 1 minute. Add broccoli and stir fry for about 2-3 minutes. Stir in cooked beef, soy sauce and lime juice and cook for about 3-4 minutes.

Serve hot.

Nutrition:

Calories: 282
Carbohydrates: 7.6g
Protein: 33.1g
Fat: 13.5g
Sugar: 2.7g
Sodium: 749mg
Fiber: 2.3g

81. Pesto Flavored Steak

Preparation Time: 15 minutes

Cooking Time: 17 minutes

Servings: 4

Ingredients:

¼ C. fresh oregano, chopped

1½ tbsp. garlic, minced

1 tbsp. fresh lemon peel, grated

½ tsp. red pepper flakes, crushed

Salt and freshly ground black pepper, to taste

1 lb. (1-inch thick) grass-fed boneless beef top sirloin steak

1 C. pesto

¼ C. feta cheese, crumbled

Direction:

Preheat the gas grill to medium heat. Lightly, grease the grill grate.

In a bowl, add the oregano, garlic, lemon peel, red pepper flakes, salt and black pepper and mix well.

Rub the garlic mixture onto the steak evenly.

Place the steak onto the grill and cook, covered for about 12-17 minutes, flipping occasionally.

Remove from the grill and place the steak onto a cutting board for about 5 minutes.

With a sharp knife, cut the steak into desired sized slices.

Divide the steak slices and pesto onto serving plates and serve with the topping of the feta cheese.

Nutrition:

Calories: 226
Carbohydrates: 6.8g
Protein: 40.5g
Fat: 7.6g
Sugar: 0.7g
Sodium: 579mg
Fiber: 2.2g

82. Flawless Grilled Steak

Preparation Time: 21 minutes

Cooking Time: 10 minutes

Servings: 5

Ingredients:

½ tsp. dried thyme, crushed

½ tsp. dried oregano, crushed

1 tsp. red chili powder

½ tsp. ground cumin

¼ tsp. garlic powder

Salt and freshly ground black pepper, to taste

1½ lb. grass-fed flank steak, trimmed

¼ C. Monterrey Jack cheese, crumbled

Direction:

In a large bowl, add the dried herbs and spices and mix well.

Add the steaks and rub with mixture generously. Set aside for about 15-20 minutes. Preheat the grill to medium heat. Grease the grill grate. Place the steak onto the grill over medium coals and cook for about 17-21 minutes, flipping once halfway through. Remove the steak from grill and place onto a cutting board for about 10 minutes before slicing. With a sharp knife, cut the steak into desired sized slices.

Top with the cheese and serve.

Nutrition:

Calories: 271
Carbohydrates: 0.7g
Protein: 38.3g
Fat: 11.8g
Sugar: 0.1g
Sodium: 119mg
Fiber: 0.3g

83. Mongolian Beef

Preparation Time: 15 minutes

Cooking Time: 10 minutes

Servings: 4

Ingredients:

1 lb. grass-fed flank steak, cut into thin slices against the grain

2 tsp. arrowroot starch

Salt, to taste

¼ C. avocado oil

1 (1-inch) piece fresh ginger, grated

4 garlic cloves, minced

½ tsp. red pepper flakes, crushed

¼ C. water

1/3 C. low-sodium soy sauce

1 tsp. red boat fish sauce

3 scallions, sliced

1 tsp. sesame seeds

Direction:

In a bowl, add the steak slices, arrowroot starch and salt and toss to coat well.

In a larger skillet, heat oil over medium-high heat and cook the steak slices for about 1½ minutes per side. With a slotted spoon, transfer the steak slices onto a plate. Drain the oil from the skillet but leaving about 1 tbsp. inside. In the same skillet, add the ginger, garlic and red pepper flakes and sauté for about 1 minute.

Add the water, soy sauce and fish sauce and stir to combine well.

Stir in the cooked steak slices and simmer for about 3 minutes.

Stir in the scallions and simmer for about 2 minutes.

Remove from the heat and serve hot with the garnishing of sesame seeds.

Nutrition:

Calories: 266
Carbohydrates: 5.7g
Protein: 34g
Fat: 11.7g
Sugar: 1.7g
Sodium: 1350mg
Fiber: 1.2g

84. Sicilian Steak Pinwheel

Preparation Time: 15 minutes

Cooking Time: 35 minutes

Servings: 6

Ingredients:

2 tbsp. dried oregano leaves

1/3 C. fresh lemon juice

2 tbsp. olive oil

1 (2-lb.) grass-fed beef flank steak, pounded into ½-inch thickness.

1/3 C. olive tapenade

1 C. frozen chopped spinach, thawed and squeezed

¼ C. feta cheese, crumbled

4 C. fresh cherry tomatoes

Salt, to taste

Direction:

In a large baking dish, add the oregano, lemon juice and oil and mix well.

Add the steak and coat with the marinade generously.

Refrigerate to marinate for about 4 hours, flipping occasionally.

Preheat the oven to 425 degrees F. Line a shallow baking dish with parchment paper.

Remove the steak from baking dish, reserving the remaining marinade in a bowl.

Cover the bowl of marinade and refrigerate.

Arrange the steak onto a cutting board.

Place the tapenade onto the steak evenly and top with the spinach, followed by the feta cheese.

Carefully, roll the steak tightly to form a log.

With 6 kitchen string pieces, tie the log at 6 places.

Carefully, cut the log between strings into 6 equal pieces, leaving string in place.

In a bowl, add the reserved marinade, tomatoes and salt and toss to coat.

Arrange the log pieces onto the prepared baking dish, cut-side up.

Now, arrange the tomatoes around the pinwheels evenly.

Bake for about 25-35 minutes.

Remove from the oven and set aside for about 5 minutes before serving.

Nutrition:

Calories: 395
Carbohydrates: 7.3g
Protein: 48.4g
Fat: 18.2g
Sugar: 3.8g
Sodium: 387mg
Fiber: 2.2g

85. American Beef Wellington

Preparation Time: 20 minutes

Cooking Time: 40 minutes

Servings: 4

Ingredients:

2 (4-oz.) grass-fed beef tenderloin steaks, halved

Salt and freshly ground black pepper, to taste

1 tbsp. butter

1 C. mozzarella cheese, shredded

½ C. almond flour

4 tbsp. liver pate

Direction:

Preheat the oven to 400 degrees F. Grease a baking sheet.

Season the steaks with salt and black pepper evenly.

In a frying pan, melt the butter over medium-high heat and sear the bee steaks for about 2-3 minutes per side.

Remove from the heat and set aside to cool completely.

Ina microwave-safe bowl, add the mozzarella cheese and microwave for about 1 minute.

Remove from the microwave and immediately, stir in the almond flour until a dough forms.

Place the dough between 2 parchment paper pieces and with a rolling pin, roll to flat it.

Remove the upper parchment paper piece.

Divide the rolled dough into 4 pieces.

Place 1 tbsp. of pate onto each dough piece and top with 1 steak piece.

Cover each steak piece with dough completely.

Arrange the covered steak pieces onto the prepared baking sheet in a single layer.

Bake for about 20-30 minutes or until the pastry is a golden brown.

Serve warm.

Nutrition:

Calories: 254
Carbohydrates: 3.9g
Protein: 19g
Fat: 16g
Sugar: 0.5g
Sodium: 410mg
Fiber: 1.5g

86. Pastry-Free Beef Wellington

Preparation Time: 20 minutes

Cooking Time: 40 minutes

Servings: 2

Ingredients:

For Duxelles:

2 tbsp. olive oil

3 large button mushrooms

1 tbsp. yellow onions, chopped

1 tsp. garlic powder

Salt, to taste

For Filling:

8 thin prosciutto slices

1 (9-oz.) grass-fed filet mignon

Salt, to taste

2 tbsp. olive oil

1 tbsp. yellow mustard

Direction:

Preheat the oven to 400 degrees F. Grease a baking sheet.

For duxelles: in a food processor, add the mushrooms,

onions, garlic, salt, and oil and pulse until pureed.

In a nonstick frying pan, add the pureed mixture over medium heat and cook for about 10 minutes, stirring frequently.

Remove from the heat and set aside.

Place a large piece of cling film onto a smooth surface.

Arrange the prosciutto slices over cling film, side-by-side form a rectangular layer, overlapping slightly.

Spread the duxelles over the prosciutto layer evenly.

Season the filet mignon with a little salt.

In a frying pan, heat the oil and sear the filet mignon fir about 2 minutes per side.

Remove from the heat and place the filet mignon onto a plate.

Now, spread the mustard over the filet mignon evenly.

Arrange the filet mignon in the middle of the prosciutto and duxelles layer.

Carefully, wrap the prosciutto around the filet mignon.

Then wrap the cling-film around the package to secure it.

With a second piece of cling film, wrap the prosciutto-wrapped package tighter and refrigerate for about 15 minutes.

Remove the cling-film from the prosciutto-wrapped beef and arrange onto the prepared baking sheet.

Bake for 20-25 minutes.

Remove from the oven and cut the beef Wellington in 2 portions.

Serve warm.

Nutrition:

Calories: 302
Carbohydrates: 2.1g
Protein: 20.1g
Fat: 20.6g
Sugar: 0.6g
Sodium: 855mg
Fiber: 0.4g

Keto Fish & Seafood Recipes

87. Super Salmon Parcel

Preparation Time: 15 minutes

Cooking Time: 20 minutes

Servings: 6

Ingredients:

6 (3-oz.) salmon fillets

Salt and freshly ground black pepper, to taste

1 yellow bell pepper, seeded and cubed

1 red bell pepper, seeded and cubed

4 plum tomatoes, cubed

1 small yellow onion, sliced thinly

½ C. fresh parsley, chopped

¼ C. olive oil

2 tbsp. fresh lemon juice

Direction:

Preheat the oven to 400 degrees F.

Arrange 6 pieces of foil onto a smooth surface. Place 1 salmon fillet onto each foil piece and sprinkle with salt and black pepper. In a bowl, add the bell peppers, tomato and onion and mix. Place veggie mixture over each fillet evenly and top with parsley. Drizzle with oil and lemon juice. Fold the foil around salmon mixture to seal it. Arrange the foil packets onto a large baking sheet in a single layer. Bake for about 20 minutes.

Serve hot.

Nutrition:

Calories: 224
Carbohydrates: 8.2g
Protein: 18.2g
Fat: 14g
Sugar: 5g
Sodium: 811mg
Fiber: 1.9g

88. New England Salmon Pie

Preparation Time: 20 minutes

Cooking Time: 50 minutes

Servings: 5

Ingredients:

For Crust:

¾ C. almond flour

4 tbsp. coconut flour

4 tbsp. sesame seeds

1 tbsp. psyllium husk powder

1 tsp. organic baking powder

Pinch of salt

1 organic egg

3 tbsp. olive oil

4 tbsp. water

For Filling:

8 oz. smoked salmon

4¼ oz. cream cheese, softened

1¼ C. cheddar cheese, shredded

1 C. mayonnaise

3 organic eggs

2 tbsp. fresh dill, finely chopped

½ tsp. onion powder

¼ tsp. ground black pepper

Direction:

Preheat the oven to 350 degrees F. Line a 10-inch spring form pan with parchment paper.

For crust: place all the ingredients in a food processor, fitted with a plastic pastry blade and pulse until a dough ball is formed.

Place the dough into prepared spring form pan and with your fingers, gently press in the bottom.

Bake for about 12-15 minutes or until lightly browned.

Remove the pie crust from oven and let it cool slightly.

Meanwhile, for filling: in a bowl add all the ingredients and mix well.

Place the cheese mixture over the pie crust evenly.

Bake for about 35 minutes or until the pie is golden brown.

Remove the pie from oven and let it cool slightly.

Cut into 5 equal-sized slices and serve warm.

Nutrition:

Calories: 762
Carbohydrates: 10.8g
Protein: 24.8g
Fat: 70g
Sugar: 0.7g
Sodium: 1500mg
Fiber: 5.3g

89. Juicy Garlic Butter Shrimp

Preparation Time: 10 minutes

Cooking Time: 5 minutes

Servings: 4

Ingredients:

2 lbs shrimp, peeled and deveined

2 tbsp fresh herbs, chopped

2 tbsp fresh lemon juice

1 tsp paprika

1 tbsp garlic, minced

1/4 cup butter

Pepper

Salt

Direction:

Melt butter in a pan over medium heat.

Add garlic and saute for 30 seconds.

Add shrimp, paprika, pepper, and salt. Cook shrimp for 2 minutes on each side.

Add remaining Ingredients and stir well and cook for 1 minute.

Serve and enjoy.

Nutrition:

Calories 379 Fat 15.5 g
Carbs:5 g
Sugar 0.3 g
Protein 52.1 g
Cholesterol 508 mg

90. Simple Lemon Garlic Shrimp

Preparation Time: 5 minutes

Cooking Time: 15 minutes

Servings: 4

Ingredients:

1 1/2 lbs shrimp, peeled and deveined

1/4 cup fresh parsley, chopped

1/4 cup fresh lemon juice

1 tbsp garlic, minced

1/4 cup butter

Pepper - Salt

Directions: Melt butter in a pan over medium heat. Add garlic and saute for 30 seconds. Add shrimp and season with pepper and salt and cook for 4-5 minutes or until it turns to pink. Add lemon juice and parsley and stir well and cook for 2 minutes. Serve and enjoy.

Nutrition: Calories 312 Fat 14.6 g
Carbs:3.9 g
Sugar 0.4 g
Protein 39.2 g
Cholesterol 389 mg

91. Flavorful Shrimp Creole

Preparation Time: 10 minutes

Cooking Time: 1 hour 30 minutes

Servings: 8

Ingredients:

2 lbs shrimp, peeled

3/4 cup green onions, chopped

1 tsp garlic, minced

2 1/2 cups water

1 tbsp hot sauce

8 oz can tomato sauce, sugar-free

8 oz can tomato paste

1/2 cup bell pepper, chopped

3/4 cup celery, chopped

1 cup onion, chopped

2 tbsp olive oil

Pepper

Salt

Direction:

Heat oil in a saucepan over medium heat.

Add celery, onion, bell pepper, pepper, and salt and saute until onion is softened.

Add tomato paste and cook for 5 minutes.

Add hot sauce, tomato sauce, and water and cook for 1 hour.

Add garlic and shrimp and cook for 15 minutes.

Add green onions and cook for 2 minutes more.

Serve and enjoy.

Nutrition:

Calories 208 Fat 5.7 g
Carbs:11.6 g
Sugar 6 g
Protein 27.9 g
Cholesterol 239 mg

92. Creamy Scallops

Preparation Time: 10 minutes

Cooking Time: 10 minutes

Servings: 4

Ingredients:

1 lb scallops, rinse and pat dry

1 tsp fresh parsley, chopped

1/8 tsp cayenne pepper

2 tbsp white wine

1/4 cup water

3 tbsp heavy cream

1 tsp garlic, minced

1 tbsp butter, melted

1 tbsp olive oil - Pepper - Salt

Direction:

Season scallops with pepper and salt. Heat butter and oil in a pan over medium heat. Add scallops and sear until browned from both the sides. Transfer scallops on a plate.

Add garlic in the same pan and saute for 30 seconds.

Add water, heavy cream, wine, cayenne pepper, and salt. Stir well and cook until sauce thickens. Return scallops to pan and stir well. Garnish with parsley and serve.

Nutrition:

Calories 202 Fat 11.4 g
Carbs:3.5 g
Sugar 0.1 g
Protein 19.4 g
Cholesterol 60 mg

93. Perfect Pan-Seared Scallops

Preparation Time: 10 minutes

Cooking Time: 4 minutes

Servings: 4

Ingredients:

1 lb scallops, rinse and pat dry

1 tbsp olive oil

2 tbsp butter

Pepper

Salt

Direction:

Season scallops with pepper and salt.

Heat butter and oil in a pan over medium heat.

Add scallops and sear for 2 minutes then turn to other side and cook for 2 minutes more.

Serve and enjoy.

Nutrition:

Calories 181 Fat 10.1 g
Carbs:2.7 g
Sugar 0 g
Protein 19.1 g
Cholesterol 53 mg

94. Easy Baked Shrimp Scampi

Preparation Time: 10 minutes

Cooking Time: 10 minutes

Servings: 4

Ingredients:

2 lbs shrimp, peeled

3/4 cup olive oil

2 tsp dried oregano

1 tbsp garlic, minced

1/2 cup fresh lemon juice

1/4 cup butter, sliced Pepper

Salt

Directions: Preheat the oven to 350 F. Add shrimp in a baking dish. In a bowl, whisk together lemon juice, oregano, garlic, oil, pepper, and salt and pour over shrimp. Add butter on top of shrimp. Bake in preheated oven for 10 minutes or until shrimp cooked. Serve and enjoy.

Nutrition:

Calories 708 Fat 53.5 g
Carbs:5.3 g Sugar 0.7 g Protein 52.2 g Cholesterol 508 mg

95. Delicious Blackened Shrimp

Preparation Time: 10 minutes

Cooking Time: 5 minutes

Servings: 4

Ingredients:

1 1/2 lbs shrimp, peeled

1 tbsp garlic, minced

1 tbsp olive oil

1 tsp garlic powder

1 tsp dried oregano

1 tsp cumin

1 tbsp paprika

1 tbsp chili powder

Pepper

Salt

Direction:

In a mixing bowl, mix together garlic powder, oregano, cumin, paprika, chili powder, pepper, and salt.

Add shrimp and mix until well coated. Set aside for 30 minutes.

Heat oil in a pan over medium-high heat.

Add shrimp and cook for 2 minutes. Turn shrimp and cook for 2 minutes more.

Add garlic and cook for 30 seconds.

Serve and enjoy.

Nutrition:

Calories 252 Fat 7.1 g
Carbs:6.3 g
Sugar 0.5 g
Protein 39.6 g
Cholesterol 358 mg

96. Creamy Parmesan Shrimp

Preparation Time: 10 minutes

Cooking Time: 20 minutes

Servings: 4

Ingredients:

1 1/2 lbs shrimp

1/2 cup chicken stock

1/4 tsp red pepper flakes

1 cup parmesan cheese, grated

1 cup fresh basil leaves

1 1/2 cups heavy cream

1/4 tsp paprika

3 oz roasted red peppers, sliced

1/2 onion, minced

1 tbsp garlic, minced

3 tbsp butter

Pepper

Salt

Direction:

Melt 2 tbsp butter in a pan over medium heat.

Season shrimp with pepper and salt and sear in a pan for 1-2 minutes. Transfer shrimp on a plate.

Add remaining butter in a pan.

Add red chili flakes, paprika, roasted peppers, garlic, onion, pepper, and salt and cook for 5 minutes.

Add stock and stir well and cook until liquid reduced by half.

Turn heat to low and add cream and stir for 1-2 minutes.

Add basil and parmesan cheese and stir for 1-2 minutes.

Return shrimp to the pan and cook for 1-2 minutes.

Serve and enjoy.

Nutrition:

Calories 524 Fat 33.2 g
Carbs:8.3 g
Sugar 1.7 g
Protein 47.8 g
Cholesterol 459 mg

97. Pan Fry Shrimp & Zucchini

Preparation Time: 10 minutes

Cooking Time: 20 minutes

Servings: 4

Ingredients:

1 lb shrimp, peeled and deveined

1/2 small onion, chopped

1 summer squash, chopped

1 zucchini, chopped

2 tbsp olive oil

1/2 tsp paprika

1/2 tsp garlic powder

1/2 tsp onion powder

Pepper

Salt

Direction:

In a large bowl, mix together paprika, garlic powder, onion powder, pepper, and salt. Add shrimp and toss well.

Heat 1 tbsp oil in a pan over medium heat,

Add shrimp and cook for 2 minutes on each side or until shrimp turns to pink. Transfer shrimp on a plate.

Add remaining oil in a pan.

Add onion, summer squash, and zucchini and cook for 6-8 minutes or until vegetables are softened.

Return shrimp to the pan and cook for 1 minute.

Serve and enjoy.

Nutrition:

Calories 215 Fat 9.1 g
Carbs:6.1 g
Sugar 2.6 g
Protein 27 g
Cholesterol 239 mg

Keto Sauces & Dressings Recipes

98. American Jack Daniel's Sauce (Keto version)

Preparation Time: 10 minutes

Cooking Time: 25 minutes

Servings: 8

Ingredients:

1 cup water

2 tsp garlic minced

1 1/2 cups of natural granulated sweetener such Stevia

2 Tbsp of hot sauce

2 Tbsp of Coconut Aminos (soy sauce substitute

1 cup of lemon juice

1/4 cup of Jack Daniels Whiskey

2 Tbsp unsalted butter

1/4 tsp cayenne pepper

Direction:

In a small saucepan, pour the water, garlic, stevia sweetener, hot sauce and Cococnut aminos.

Cook and stir over moderate heat for about 15-20 minutes until sweetener dissolve, and the sauce thickens.

Remove from heat and add the lemon juice, whiskey, butter and cayenne pepper stir well until sauce is smooth and shine.

Let it cool and keep refrigerated in a glass container up to 3 months.

Nutrition:

Calories: 61 Carbohydrates: 5g Proteins: 1g Fat: 4g Fiber: 0.2g

99. Fresh Mushroom Sauce

Preparation Time: 10 minutes

Cooking Time: 15 minutes

Servings: 6

Ingredients:

1/4 cup of garlic-infused olive oil

1 tsp of garlic minced

1 lbs. fresh white mushrooms, sliced

1 cup of cherry tomatoes, cut into halves

1/2 cup green onions (scallions finely chopped

1/2 tsp salt and ground black pepper to taste

Direction:

Heat the olive oil in a frying skillet.

Add minced garlic along with mushrooms, and cook, stirring frequently, until mushroom liquid starts to evaporate, about 5 - 6 minutes.

Add cherry tomatoes, green onions, and season with the salt and black pepper.

Bring to boil, reduce heat, cover and cook for about 5 minutes or until the sauce is done.

Remove from heat and serve hot or cold.

Keep refrigerated in a covered glass bowl.

Nutrition:

Calories: 105 Carbohydrates: 4g Proteins: 3g Fat: 10g Fiber: 1.3g

100. Spicy Citrus BBQ Sauce

Preparation Time: 10 minutes

Cooking Time: 15 minutes

Servings: 6

Ingredients:

2 Tbsp of olive oil

1 large onion finely chopped

1/2 tsp ground red pepper (cayenne

1 chili pepper, seeded and finely chopped

1 1/2 cups lime juice (freshly squeezed

2 Tbsp of stevia granulate sweetener (or to taste

1 Tbsp of fresh cilantro finely chopped

1/4 tsp salt or to taste

Direction:

Heat the olive oil in a saucepan, and cook the onion, ground red pepper, and chili pepper, stirring frequently, until onion is tender, about 5 minutes. At this point, add all remaining Ingredients.

Bring to boil and reduce heat to the low cook for further 10 minutes, stirring occasionally.

Remove the sauce from heat and allow it to cool.

Serve immediately or keep refrigerated.

Nutrition:

Calories: 61 Carbohydrates: 6g Proteins: 1g Fat: 5g Fiber: 0.7g

101. Italian Pesto Dip with Ground Almonds

Preparation Time: 10 minutes

Cooking Time: 0 Minutes

Servings: 4

Ingredients:

2 cup of fresh basil

2 cloves of garlic minced

3 Tbsp of ground almonds, salted

3/4 cup extra virgin olive oil

1 Tbsp of lemon juice

Salt and ground black pepper

4 Tbsp of ground Parmesan cheese

Direction: Place all Ingredients (except Parmesan in a food processor and pulse until well combined. Add the parmesan cheese and pulse for 30 - 45 seconds. Taste and adjust salt and pepper to taste. Keep refrigerated.

Nutrition:

Calories: 426 Carbohydrates: 3g Proteins: 4g Fat: 45g Fiber: 1g

102. Keto "Chimichurri" Sauce

Preparation Time: 10 minutes

Cooking Time: 0 Minutes

Servings: 6

Ingredients:

1/2 cup of fresh oregano leaves, finely chopped

1/2 cup of fresh parsley, finely chopped

1/2 cup fresh cilantro, finely chopped

3 fresh bay leaves

2 jalapenos peppers, chopped

3 cloves garlic

1 Tbsp salt

1 Tbsp of chili powder

1/2 cup apple cider vinegar

1/2 cup of olive oil

Direction:

Add Ingredients from the list above in your food processor or blender.

Blend or process until smooth and all Ingredients are united well.

Serve immediately or keep refrigerated.

Nutrition:

Calories: 201 Carbohydrates: 8g Proteins: 1.2g Fat: 19g Fiber: 4g

Keto Smoothies Recipes

103. Peanut butter cup smoothie

Preparation Time: 5 minutes

Cooking Time: 0 Minutes

Servings: 2

Ingredients:

1 cup water

¾ cup coconut cream

1 scoop chocolate protein powder

2 tablespoons natural peanut butter

3 ice cubes

Direction:

Put the water, coconut cream, protein powder, peanut butter, and ice in a blender and blend until smooth.

Pour into 2 glasses and serve immediately.

Nutrition:

Calories: 486
Fat: 40g
Protein: 30g
Carbs: 11g
Fiber: 5g
Net Carbs: 6g
Fat 70%/Protein 20%/Carbs 10%

104. Berry green smoothie

Preparation Time: 10 minutes

Cooking Time: 0 Minutes

Servings: 2

Ingredients:

1 cup water

½ cup raspberries

½ cup shredded kale

¾ cup cream cheese

1 tablespoon coconut oil

1 scoop vanilla protein powder

Direction:

Put the water, raspberries, kale, cream cheese, coconut oil, and protein powder in a blender and blend until smooth.

Pour into 2 glasses and serve immediately.

Nutrition:

Calories: 436
Fat: 36g
Protein: 28g
Carbs: 11g
Fiber: 5g
Net Carbs: 6g
Fat 70%/Protein 20%/Carbs 10%

105. Lemon-cashew smoothie

Preparation Time: 5 minutes

Cooking Time: 0 Minutes

Servings: 1

Ingredients:

1 cup unsweetened cashew milk

¼ cup heavy (whipping) cream

¼ cup freshly squeezed lemon juice

1 scoop plain protein powder

1 tablespoon coconut oil

1 teaspoon sweetener

Direction:

Put the cashew milk, heavy cream, lemon juice, protein powder, coconut oil, and sweetener in a blender and blend until smooth.

Pour into a glass and serve immediately.

Nutrition:

Calories: 503
Fat: 45g
Protein: 29g
Carbs: 15g
Fiber: 4g
Net Carbs: 11g
Fat 80%/Protein 13%/Carbs 7%

106. Spinach-blueberry smoothie

Preparation Time: 5 minutes

Cooking Time: 0 Minutes

Servings: 2

Ingredients: 1 cup spinach

1 cup coconut milk

½ English cucumber, chopped

½ cup blueberries

1 scoop plain protein powder

2 tablespoons coconut oil

4 ice cubes

Mint sprigs, for garnish

Direction:

Put the coconut milk, spinach, cucumber, blueberries, protein powder, coconut oil, and ice in a blender and blend until smooth. Pour into 2 glasses, garnish each with the mint, and serve immediately.

Nutrition: Calories:353 Fat:32g Protein:15g Carbs:9g Fiber:3g NetCarbs:6g Fat76%/Protein16%/Carbs 8%

107. Creamy cinnamon smoothie

Preparation Time: 5 minutes

Cooking Time: 0 Minutes

Servings: 2

Ingredients:

2 cups coconut milk

1 scoop vanilla protein powder

5 drops liquid stevia

1 teaspoon ground cinnamon

½ teaspoon alcohol-free vanilla extract

Direction:

Put the coconut milk, protein powder, stevia, cinnamon, and vanilla in a blender and blend until smooth. Pour into 2 glasses and serve immediately.

Nutrition: Calories: 492
Fat: 47g
Protein: 18g
Carbs: 8g
Fiber: 2g
Net Carbs: 6g
Fat 80%/Protein 14%/Carbs 6%

Keto Vegan Recipes

108. Chocolate Sea Salt Smoothie

Preparation Time: 5 minutes

Cooking Time: 0 Minutes

Servings: 2

Ingredients:

1 avocado (frozen or not)

2 cups almond milk

1 tbsp tahini

¼ cup cocoa powder

1 scoop perfect Keto chocolate base

Direction: Combine all the ingredients in a high speed blender and mix until you get a soft smoothie. Add ice and enjoy!

Nutrition:

Calories: 235 calories, 20g fat, 11.25 carbohydrates, 8g fiber, and 5.5g protein

109. Eggplant Lasagna

Preparation Time: 20 minutes

Cooking Time: 1 hour 10 minutes

Servings: 6

Ingredients:

1 Eggplant, large and sliced into thin rounds

1 TBSP Salt

1 C Marinara Sauce, low carb

.5 C Vegan Cheese, shredded

1 C Vegan Ricotta

Some Olive Oil

Direction:

Lay eggplant rounds in a single layer on a tray and liberally salt the slices, then flip them over and salt the other sides. Let stand for 1 hour so moisture beads up on the surface. Rinse the eggplant rounds and press them dry, as this will help you get out as much moisture as possible.

Turn your oven on to 350F. Brush a modest layer of olive oil over the bottom of an 8x8 baking dish, then make a single layer of eggplant rounds. Lightly layer marinara sauce over the eggplant layer, then top the layer with half of your vegan cheese shreds. Create another layer of eggplant rounds, then cover that layer with vegan ricotta and a thin layer of marinara sauce. Place one final layer of eggplant rounds on your lasagna, then spread the rest of your marinara sauce on the eggplant and the remaining vegan cheese on the sauce layer.

Bake your eggplant lasagna for 30 minutes, covered. Then, bake uncovered for an additional 15 minutes. Let it cool for 10 minutes before serving your eggplant lasagna.

Nutrition:

427kcal

110. Keto Vegan Cauliflower and Tofu Stir Fry

Preparation Time: 15 minutes

Cooking Time: 15 minutes

Servings: 4

Ingredients:

14 OZ Tofu, extra firm

1.5 TBSP Sesame Oil

1 Head Cauliflower, small cut into florets

2 Cloves Garlic, minced

.25 C Soy Sauce, low sodium

.5 TSP Chili Garlic Sauce

2.5 TBSP Peanut Butter, natural and salted

Direction:

Drain and press your tofu about 1.5 hours before you are ready to start preparing your stir fry so that it is completely dry when you start. When it is dry, cube it into 1" cubes. Turn your oven on to 400F. Cook tofu cubes for 25 minutes, then remove it from the oven and let your tofu cool down as you prepare the rest of your recipe. Whisk together sesame oil, soy sauce, chili garlic sauce, and peanut butter to prepare a marinade and let your tofu soak in it for 15 minutes so that it absorbs the flavor of the sauce. Place your cauliflower in a food processor or blender and pulse until it resembles cauliflower rice.

Heat excess marinade in a pan over the oven and then add the tofu and brown the edges of your tofu. Then, set them aside and heat your cauliflower rice in the excess sauce. The rice should cook for approximately 5-8 minutes, until it is slightly browned and tender.

Serve your tofu over your cauliflower rice right away using any leftover sauce, you may have to add even more flavor. Store leftovers in the fridge for up to 3 days, using a pan to reheat them when you are ready to eat more.

Nutrition:

Calories: 297, Fat: 15.6g, Protein: 21.1g, Cholesterol 139.5mg

111. Keto Vegan Curry

Preparation Time: 15 minutes

Cooking Time: 20 minutes

Servings: 4

Ingredients:

.25 C Vegan Butter

4 TBSP Coconut Oil, melted

16 OZ Tofu, extra firm and cubed

1 C Baby Spinach

1 Carrot, diced

1 Zucchini, diced

.5 Bell Pepper, sliced thin

2 Garlic Cloves, sliced thin

2.5 TBSP Vegan Red Curry Paste

1 C Vegetable Stock

1.5 C Coconut Milk, unsweetened and full fat

2 TBSP Peanut Butter, natural and unsweetened

2 TBSP Vegan Protein Powder, flavorless

4 Drops Liquid Stevia

.25 C Fresh Cilantro, chopped

1 TSP Salt

1 TSP Black Pepper

Direction:

Melt vegan butter over medium heat in a large stock pot. Add bell pepper and garlic and warm for about 1 minute, then add your curry paste. Stir constantly for 1 minute before adding your carrot, zucchini, coconut milk, protein powder, vegetable stock, stevia, peanut butter, and salt and pepper. Continue stirring until all ingredients are properly blended together.

Boil, then reduce your curry to a simmer and cook uncovered for about 8-10 minutes, until all of the vegetables are tender. Adjust your seasoning to your taste preferences.

Toss tofu cubes into the curry and simmer for an additional 5 minutes, so they are completely warmed all the way through, then add your spinach and cilantro, so they have time to wilt into the soup.

Serve coconut curry into four serving bowls and drizzle each bowl with 1 TBSP of the melted coconut oil.

Nutrition: 425 calories, 33g fat, 18g protein, 10g carbs, 2g sugars

112. Shirataki Noodles With Vegan Alfredo Sauce

Preparation Time: 10 minutes

Cooking Time: 15 minutes

Servings: 4

Ingredients:

1 Package Shirataki Noodles

1 Bag Cauliflower Rice

1 TBSP Lemon Juice

2 TBSP Avocado Oil

4 Cloves Garlic, minced

1.5 C Almond Milk, plain and unsweetened

1.5 C Cashews, soaked for at least 4 hours then drained

3 TBSP Nutritional Yeast

Direction:

Cook your shirataki noodles according to the instructions on the package.

Microwave cauliflower rice according to bag instructions, then remove to let the bag cool.

Warm avocado oil and minced garlic in a pan over medium heat until fragrant, then add the garlic mix, cauliflower rice, soaked cashews, almond milk, nutritional yeast, and lemon juice to a blender and blend it until smooth.

Pour your sauce back into the pan and add your cooked shirataki noodles and cook for about 7 minutes, until everything is warmed and well blended.

Serve.

Nutrition:

340 calories

Keto Chaffle Recipes

113. Peanut chaffles

Preparation Time: 5 minutes

Cooking Time: 5 minutes

Servings: 1

Ingredients:

- 1 egg
- 1/2 cup shredded mozzarella cheese
- 1 Tablespoon finely ground peanuts

Direction:

Preheat waffle iron.

In a little bowl, whisk the one egg and the cheddar with a fork until consolidated.

For a peanut waffle chaffle, include 1 Tablespoon finely ground peanuts. Blend well.

Spread a portion of the blend equally in the waffle well.

Cook for 3-4 minutes or until brilliant dark-colored. Evacuate to a plate to cool. Rehash with the residual hitter.

Nutrition:

363 Calories, 29.1g Fat, 22.6g Protein, 5.2g Net Carbs

114. Grilled cheese chaffle

Preparation Time: 3 minutes

Cooking Time: 8 minutes

Servings: 1

Ingredients:

1 egg

1/4 teaspoon garlic powder

1/2 cup shred cheddar

2 american cheese or 1/4 cup shredded cheese

1 tablespoon butter

Direction:

Preheat waffle iron.

In a small bowl, mix bacon, garlic powder and shredded cheddar cheese.

After heating the dash waffle maker, add half the mixture of the scramble. Cook and cook for 4 minutes.

Add to the dash mini waffle maker the remainder of the scramble mixture and cook for 4 minutes.

Steam the stove pan over moderate heat when both chaffles are finished.

Attach 1 spoonful of butter and dissolve. Place one chaffle in the pan once the butter has melted. Place your favorite cheese on top of the chaffle and finish with a second chaffle.

Cook the chaffle for 1 minute on the first side, turn it over and cook for another 1-2 minutes on the other side to finish the cheese melting.

Cut it from the bread when the cheese melts and eat it!

Nutrition:

Calories: 549kcal
Carbohydrates: 3g, Protein: 27g, Fats: 48g, Saturated fats: 28g,Cholesterol: 295mg,Sodium: 1216mg,Potassium: 172mg,Sugar 1g,

115. Baked potato chaffle using jicama

Preparation Time: 5 minutes

Cooking Time: 10 minutes

Servings: 1

Ingredients:

1 jicama root

1/2 onion, medium, minced

2 cloves garlic, pressed

1 cup cheese

1 eggs, whisked

Salt and pepper

Direction:

Peel the jicama root and shred it using a food processor.

Place the shredded jicama root in a colander to allow the water to drain. Mix in 2 tsp of salt as well.

Squeeze out the remaining liquid. Microwave the shredded jicama for 5-8 minutes. This step pre-cooks it. Mix all the remaining Ingredients together with the jicama. Start preheating the waffle maker.

Once preheated, sprinkle a bit of cheese on the waffle maker, allowing it to toast for a few seconds.

Place 3 tbsp of the jicama mixture onto the waffle maker. Sprinkle more cheese on top before closing the lid.

Cook for 5 minutes. Flip the chaffle and let it cook for 2 more minutes.

Servings your baked jicama by topping it with sour cream, cheese, bacon pieces, and chives.

Nutrition:

Calories: 168
Carbohydrates: 5.1g, Fat: 11.8g, Protein: 10g

116. Breakfast chaffle sandwich

Preparation Time: 5 minutes

Cooking Time: 5 minutes

Servings: 1

Ingredients:

1 egg

1/2 cup monterey jack chee se

1 tbsp almond flour

2 tbsp butter

Direction:

Preheat the waffle maker for 5 minutes until it's hot.

Combine monterey jack cheese, almond flour, and the egg in a bowl. Mix well.

Take 1/2 of the batter and pour it into the preheated waffle maker. Allow to cook for 3-4 minutes.

Repeat previous step for the remaining batter.

Melt butter on a small pan. Just like you would with french toast, add the chaffles and let each side cook for 2 minutes. To make them crispier, press down on the chaffles while they cook.

Remove the chaffles from the pan. Allow to cool for a few minutes. Servings.

Nutrition:

Calories: 514
Carbohydrates: 2g, Fat: 47g, Protein: 21g

117. Peanut Butter and Jelly Chaffles

Preparation Time: 5 minutes

Cooking Time: 5 minutes

Servings: 1

Ingredients:

1 egg

2 slices cheese, thinly sliced

1 tsp natural peanut butter

1 tsp sugar-free raspberr y preServings

Cooking spray

Direction:

Crack and whisk the egg in a small bowl or a measuring cup.

Lightly grease the waffle maker with Cooking spray.

Preheat the waffle maker.

Once it is heated up, place a slice of cheese on the waffle maker and wait for it to melt.

Once melted, pour the egg mixture onto the melted cheese.

Once the egg starts cooking, carefully place another slice of cheese on the waffle maker.

Close the lid. Cook for 3-4 minutes.

Take out the chaffles and place on a plate.

Top the chaffles with whipped cream.

Drizzle some natural peanut butter and raspberry preServings on top.

Nutrition:

Calories: 337
Carbohydrates: 3g, Fat: 27g

118. Halloumi cheese chaffles

Preparation Time: 5 minutes

Cooking Time: 3-6 minutes

Servings: 1

Ingredients:

3 oz halloumi cheese

2 tbsp pasta sauce

Direction:

Make half-inch thick slices of halloumi cheese.

With the waffle maker still turned off, place the cheese slices on it.

Turn on the waffle maker and let the cheese cook for 3-6 minutes.

Remove from the waffle maker and let it cool.

Add low-carb pasta or marinara sauce.

Nutrition:

Calories: 333
Carbohydrates: 2g, Fat: 26g, Protein: 22g

119. Chaffles benedict

Preparation Time: 15 minutes

Cooking Time: 10 minutes

Servings: 4

Ingredients:

12 eggs

1 cup cheddar cheese, shredded

8 slices bacon

3 egg yolks

1 tbsp lemon juice

2 pinches kosher salt

1/4 tsp dijon mustard or hot sauce, optional

1/2 cup butter, salted

Direction:

Preheat the waffle maker.

Pour water in a pan and place over medium-high heat.

Take 4 eggs and beat them in a bowl. The remaining eggs are for poaching.

Once the waffle maker is heated up, sprinkle 1 tbsp of cheese and allow it to toast.

Take 1 1/2 tbsp of the beaten eggs and place on the toasted cheese.

Once the egg starts cooking, add another layer of sprinkled cheese on top.

Close the lid. Cook for 2-3 minutes.

Remove the cooked chaffle and repeat the steps until you've created 8 chaffles.

Fry bacon and set aside for later.

Poach the remaining eggs.

To make the sauce, combine lemon juice, salt, egg yolks, and dijon mustard or hot sauce in a bowl.

In a separate container, melt the butter in the microwave. Let it cool for a few minutes.

Pour the melted butter over the egg yolk mixture.

Using an immersion blender, pulse the mixture until it becomes yellow and cloudy. Continue pulsing until the consistency becomes creamy and thick.

To Servings, place cooked chaffles on a plate.

Place a slice of bacon over each chaffle.

Top the bacon with poached egg and drizzle with hollandaise sauce.

Nutrition:

Calories: 601
Carbohydrates: 1g, Fat: 51g, Protein: 34g

120. Eggnog chaffles

Preparation Time: 5 minutes

Cooking Time: 5 minutes

Servings: 1

Ingredients:

1 egg, separated

1 egg yolk

1/2 cup mozzarella che ese, shredded

1/2 tsp spiced rum

1 tsp vanilla extract

1/4 tsp nutmeg, dried

A dash of cinnamon

1 tsp coconut flour

2 tbsp cream cheese

1 tbsp powdered sweetener

2 tsp rum or rum extract

Direction:

Preheat the mini waffle maker.

Mix egg yolk in a small bowl until smooth.

Add in the sweetener and mix until the powder is completely dissolved.

Add the coconut flour, cinnamon, and nutmeg. Mix well.

In another bowl, mix rum, egg white, and vanilla. Whisk until well combined.

Throw in the yolk mixture with the egg white mixture. You should be able to form a thin batter.

Add the mozzarella cheese and combine with the mixture.

Separate the batter into two batches. Put 1/2 of the batter into the waffle maker and let it cook for 6 minutes until it's solid.

Repeat until you've used up the remaining batter.

In a separate bowl, mix all the icing Ingredients.

Top the cooked chaffles with the icing, or you can use this as a dip.

Nutrition:

Calories: 266
Carbohydrates: 2g, Fat: 23g, Protein: 13g

121. Blue cheese chaffle bites

Preparation Time: 10 minutes

Cooking Time: 14 minutes

Servings: 2

Ingredients:

1 egg, beaten

½ cup finely grated parmesan cheese

¼ cup crumbled blue cheese

1 tsp erythritol

Direction:

Preheat the waffle iron.

Mix all the Ingredients in a bowl.

Open the iron and add half of the mixture. Close and cook until crispy, 7 minutes.

Remove the chaffle onto a plate and make another with the remaining mixture.

Cut each chaffle into wedges and Servings afterward.

Nutrition:

Calories 196, Fats 13.91g, Carbs 4.03g, Net carbs 4.03g, Protein 13.48g

122. Chaffle fruit snacks

Preparation Time: 10 minutes

Cooking Time: 14 minutes

Servings: 2

Ingredients:

1 egg, beaten

½ cup finely grated cheddar cheese

½ cup greek yogurt for topping

8 raspberries and blackberries for topping

Direction:

Preheat the waffle iron.

Mix the egg and cheddar cheese in a medium bowl.

Open the iron and add half of the mixture. Close and cook until crispy, 7 minutes.

Remove the chaffle onto a plate and make another with the remaining mixture.

Cut each chaffle into wedges and arrange on a plate.

Top each waffle with a tablespoon of yogurt and then two berries.

Servings afterward.

Nutrition:

Calories 207, Fats 15.29g, Carbs 4.36g, Net carbs 3.86g, Protein 12.91g

123. Keto belgian sugar chaffles

Preparation Time: 10 minutes

Cooking Time: 24 minutes

Servings: 4

Ingredients:

1 egg, beaten

2 tbsp swerve brown sugar

½ tbsp butter, melted

1 tsp vanilla extract

1 cup finely grated parmesan cheese

Direction:

Preheat the waffle iron.

Mix all the Ingredients in a medium bowl.

Open the iron and pour in a quarter of the mixture. Close and cook until crispy, 6 minutes.

Remove the chaffle onto a plate and make 3 more with the remaining Ingredients.

Cut each chaffle into wedges, plate, allow cooling and Servings.

Nutrition:

Calories 136, Fats 9.45g, Carbs 3.69g, Net carbs 3.69g, Protein 8.5g

Keto Dessert Recipes

124. No-Bake Chocolate "Oatmeal" Bars

Preparation Time: 15 minutes

Cooking Time: 10 minutes

Servings: 16

Ingredients:

Crust Ingredients:

1 cup of chopped almonds

1 cup of unsweetened coconut flakes

½ cup of granulated Erythritol-based Sweetener

1 tsp. of yacón Syrup (optional)

1 stick (½ cup) of unsalted butter

¼ tsp. of salt

100g (1 cup) blanched almond flour

½ tsp. of Vanilla extract

Filling Ingredients:

1¼ cups of heavy Whipping Cream

4 oz. finely chopped unsweetened chocolate

2 tbsp. of unsalted Butter

Direction:

Preparing the Crust:

With parchment paper, cover a 9-inch baking pan.

Process the sliced almonds and coconut in a food processor until they appear like grains of oatmeal. Set aside.

Add the vanilla extract, yacón syrup, sweetener, and butter over medium heat in a medium saucepan and thoroughly whisk to mix well. Remove from heat.

Add the almonds, salt, almond flour and coconut. Stir well. Place about two-thirds of the mixture in the baking pan.

To Make the Filling and Assemble:

Allow the cream to simmer over medium heat. Remove from heat and add the butter and chopped chocolate. Allow to melt for four minutes.

Add the vanilla extract and sweetener. Whisk the mixture until smooth.

Pour the filling on top of the crust. Sprinkle the rest of the crust mixture on top and refrigerate for 1 hour to firm up.

Remove the parchment paper and slice into 16 bars.

Nutrition:

Fat: 25.5g | Carbs: 6.5g | Protein: 4.4g | Erythritol: 15g | Fiber: 3.2g | Calories: 275

125. No-Bake Peanut Butter Caramel Cookies

Preparation Time: 5 minutes

Cooking Time: 10 minutes

Servings: 16

Ingredients:

¾ cup of creamy, salted Peanut Butter

1 cup Caramel Sauce

½ Vanilla extract or tsp Caramel

¾ cup of sliced Almonds

¾ cup unsweetened Flaked Coconut

¼ cup powdered Erythritol-based Sweetener

3 oz. of finely crushed Pork Rinds

Direction:

Line the baking sheet using parchment or wax paper.

Stir the peanut butter and the caramel over low heat in a saucepan until smooth and melted. Stir the extract and remove from heat after stirring.

Pulse the sliced almonds and flaked coconut together in a food processor until the mixture appears like an oatmeal.

Add the almond mixture and coconut plus the sweetener, and

crushed pork rinds. Stir to incorporate.

Using rounded tbsp., drop the mixture on the top of a coated baking sheet. Leave 2 inches in between them. Use palm to flatten the cookies.

Place in the refrigerator for an hour to firm.

Nutrition:

Fat: 16.6g | Carbs: 5.1g | Protein: 7.3g | Erythritol: 9.4g | Fiber: 1.7g | Calories: 200

126. Sugar Cookie Bars

Preparation Time: 15 minutes

Cooking Time: 18 minutes

Servings: 16

Ingredients:

Bar Ingredients:

2 tbsp. of Coconut flour

200g (2 cups) blanched Almond flour

½ cup of granulated Erythritol-based Sweetener

½ tsp. of baking powder

½ tsp. of Vanilla extract

1 large egg

¼ tsp. of salt

1 stick (½ cup) unsalted Butter, melted

Vanilla Frosting:

¼ cup (2 oz.) of softened Cream Cheese

½ cup (1 stick) of unsalted Butter

½ cup powdered Erythritol-based Sweetener

2-4 tbsp. of heavy Whipping Cream kept at room temp

½ tsp. of Vanilla extract

1 tbsp. of Coconut Sprinkles

Direction:

Preparing the Bars:

Heat the oven to 325°F and grease a nine-inch baking pan.

Whisk the baking powder, salt, sweetener, vanilla extract egg, and butter in a large bowl until it is well mixed.

Evenly spread the dough in greased baking pan and Bake for 18 minutes until the sides appear golden brown. At this point the middle will remain soft. Take out of the oven and allow to completely cool in the pan.

Preparing the Assemble and Frosting:

Beat in cream cheese and butter using an electric mixer in a medium bowl until smooth. Add the powdered sweetener and beat.

Add 1 tbsp. of the heavy cream until frosting becomes spreadable. Beat in the vanilla extract until well incorporated.

Evenly spread frosting on the top of the cookie and make sure to garnish with coconut sprinkles. Slice into 16 bars.

Nutrition:

Fat: 20.5g | Carbs: 3.9g | Protein: 3.9g | Erythritol: 15g | Fiber: 1.8g | Calories: 218

127. Dairy-Free Peanut Butter Bars

Preparation Time: 15 minutes

Cooking Time: 5 minutes

Servings: 16

Ingredients:

Bar Ingredients:

2 tbsp. plus ½ cup of coconut oil

¾ cup of salted Creamy Peanut Butter

⅔ cup of powdered Erythritol-based Sweetener

1 tsp Vanilla extract

200g (2 cups) of defatted Peanut flour

Chocolate Glaze Ingredients:

3 oz. of sugarless dark chopped Chocolate

1 tbsp. of Coconut oil

Direction:

Preparing the Bars:

Line a 9-inch baking pan using parchment paper.

Mix the coconut oil and peanut butter in a large bowl. Thoroughly whisk the mixture until smooth. Stir in vanilla extract and sweetener until it becomes thoroughly mixed.

Add the peanut flour and stir so that the dough sticks close. Firmly press the dough and evenly flatten it on a coated baking pan. Cover with parchment or wax paper.

Preparing the Assemble and Glaze:

Place the coconut oil and the chocolate in a microwaveable bowl. In 30-second increments, microwave on high power until smooth and melted.

Pour the glaze on the top of the bars and with a knife, spread it to the sides. Refrigerate for about an hour so that the chocolate becomes set.

Cut into sixteen bars.

Nutrition:

Fat: 19g | Carbs: 7.2g | Protein: 5.5g | Erythritol: 11g | Fiber: 2.9g | Calories: 211

128. Vanilla Bean Semifreddo

Preparation Time: 10 minutes

Cooking Time: 7 minutes

Servings: 3

Ingredients:

3 large egg yolks

2 large eggs

⅔ cup powdered Erythritol-based Sweetener

½ cup of Vanilla Beans

½ tsp Vanilla extract

1⅓ cups heavy Whipping Cream

Direction:

Set a pan over a heatproof bowl and place the 2 large eggs, 3 egg yolks and ⅓ cup of the sweetener in water that is barely simmering. For 5-7 minutes, whisk the mixture of the egg yolk and the egg until it becomes thick. Take the bowl out of the pan and allow to cool while continuing to whisk it.

If you are using vodka, whisk it in. Cut open the vanilla bean and remove its seed with a sharp knife. Stir in the vanilla seeds.

Whip the cream plus the vanilla extract and the rest of the sweetener using an electric beater until mixture holds stiff peaks. Add the egg mixture and fold it gently until no streaks remain.

Transfer the mixture to an airtight container and freeze until firm, 6 to 8 hours.

Nutrition:

Macros: Fat: 20.5g | Carbs: 3.9g | Protein: 3.9g | Erythritol: 15g | Fiber: 1.8g | Calories: 218

Conclusion

Now that you are familiar with the Keto diet on many levels, you should feel confident in your ability to start your own Keto journey. This diet plan isn't going to hinder you or limit you, so do your best to keep this in mind as you begin changing your lifestyle and adjusting your eating habits. Packed with good fats and plenty of protein, your body is going to go through a transformation as it works to see these things as energy. Before you know it, your body will have an automatically accessible reserve that you can utilize at any time. Whether you need a boost of energy first thing in the morning or a second wind to keep you going throughout the day, this will already be inside of you.

As you take care of yourself through the next few years, you can feel great knowing that the Keto diet aligns with the anti-aging lifestyle that you seek. Not only does it keep you looking great and feeling younger, but it also acts as a preventative barrier from various ailments and conditions. The body tends to weaken as you age, but Keto helps to keep a shield up in front of it by giving you plenty of opportunities to burn energy and create muscle mass. Instead of taking the things that you need in order to feel great, Keto only takes what you have in abundance. This is how you will always end up feeling your best each day.

Arguably one of the best diets around, Keto keeps you feeling so great because you have many meal options! There is no shortage of delicious and filling meals that you can eat while you are on any of the Keto diet plans. You can even take this diet with you as you eat out at restaurants and at friends' houses. As long as you can remember the simple guidelines, you should have no problems staying on track with Keto. Cravings become almost non-existent as your body works to change the way it digests. Instead of relying on glucose in your bloodstream, your body switches focus. It begins using fat as soon as you reach the state of ketosis that you are aiming for. The best part is, you do not have to do anything other than eating within your fat/protein/carb percentages. Your body will do the rest on its own.

Because this is a way that your body can properly function for long periods of time, Keto is proven to be more than a simple fad diet. Originating with a medical background for helping epilepsy patients, the Keto diet has been tried and tested for decades. Many successful studies align with the knowledge that Keto really works. Whether you are trying to be on the diet for a month or a year, both are just as healthy for you. Keto is an adjustment, but it is one that will continue benefiting you for as long as you are able to keep it up. If you are ready to feel great and look great from the inside out, you can begin your Keto journey with the confidence that it is truly going to make a difference in your life. The natural signs of aging and hormonal imbalances of being a woman are not enough to hold you back when you are actively participating in a balanced Keto diet.

Change your life today and enjoy the many benefits of a Keto diet.

Printed in Great Britain
by Amazon